T0211292

The Psychology of Aphasia

of Aphasia

A Practical Guide for Health Care Professionals

The Psychology of Aphasia

A Practical Guide for Health Care Professionals

Dennis C. Tanner, PhD
Professor Emeritus
Northern Arizona University
Flagstaff, Arizona

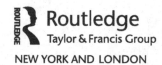

Routledge
Taylor & Francis Group

NEW YORK AND LONDON

Dr. Dennis C. Tanner has no financial or proprietary interest in the materials presented herein.

First published 2017 by SLACK Incorporated

Published 2024 by Routledge
605 Third Avenue, New York, NY 10158

and by Routledge
4 Park Square, Milton Park, Abingdon, Oxon, OX14 4RN

Routledge is an imprint of the Taylor & Francis Group, an informa business

Copyright © 2017 Taylor & Francis Group

All rights reserved. No part of this book may be reprinted or reproduced or utilised in any form or by any electronic, mechanical, or other means, now known or hereafter invented, including photocopying and recording, or in any information storage or retrieval system, without permission in writing from the publishers.

Trademark Notice: Product or corporate names may be trademarks or registered trademarks, and are used only for identification and explanation without intent to infringe.

Library of Congress Cataloging-in-Publication Data

Names: Tanner, Dennis C., 1949- author.
Title: The psychology of aphasia : a practical guide for health care
   professionals / Dennis C. Tanner.
Description: Thorofare, NJ : SLACK Incorporated, [2017] | Includes
   bibliographical references.
Identifiers: LCCN 2017002667 (print) | ISBN 9781630912680 (pbk. : alk. paper)
Subjects: | MESH: Aphasia--psychology | Aphasia--physiopathology | Disabled
   Persons--psychology
Classification: LCC RC425 (print) | NLM WL 340.5 | DDC
   616.85/52--dc23
LC record available at https://lccn.loc.gov/2017002667

ISBN: 9781630912680 (pbk)
ISBN: 9781003526049 (ebk)

DOI: 10.4324/9781003526049

DEDICATION

This book is dedicated to my grandchildren: Camden, Paxton, Elliot, and Hannah Beth.

DEDICATION

CONTENTS

ACKNOWLEDGMENTS

The author gratefully acknowledges the following people at SLACK, Incorporated for their professional help in creating this book: Brien Cummings, Jennifer Kilpatrick, Michelle Gatt, and Erin O'Reilly.

ABOUT THE AUTHOR

Dennis C. Tanner received his Doctor of Philosophy degree in Audiology and Speech Sciences from Michigan State University. He is a prolific author of books, diagnostic tests, and treatment programs. Dr. Tanner is the owner of Tanner Rehabilitation Services, Inc., a provider of speech and hearing services in Arizona for 40 years. He serves as an expert witness in legal cases involving communication sciences and disorders. Dr. Tanner is currently Professor Emeritus of Health Sciences at Northern Arizona University and was named "Outstanding Educator" by the Association of Schools of Allied Health Professions and the "Teacher of the Year" for the College of Health Professions. He is also an honorary professor at Tehran University of Medical Sciences, Tehran, Iran. Visit his website: http://www.drdennistanner.com

FOREWORD

"Yay, I had a stroke." That was my flippant reply to the wonderful intensive care unit nurse who asked me if I needed to take anything or see anyone for depression. I had just survived a left pontine cerebrovascular accident—a brainstem stroke—that had left me with severe right side hemiparesis, ataxic dysarthria, and dysphagia (Goldfarb, 2015, 2016). But not aphasia. The rigorous therapeutic road back to walking, balancing, using my right arm and hand, speaking clearly, and swallowing safely would have been magnitudes more difficult if recovering language skills was also involved.

Professor Tanner's book addresses a critical lack in the literature on recovery from aphasia. The reader must look elsewhere for a thorough review of cognitive-psycholinguistic aspects of aphasia and related disorders, but that is not the focus of this volume. Instead, Professor Tanner addresses the overwhelming disorientation that aphasia can cause in the patient, the communication partner, the communication between them, and their shared environment.

This volume is a logical expansion of an essay Professor Tanner wrote for a book I edited on *Translational Speech-Language Pathology and Audiology* (Tanner, 2012, pp. 301-306). He joined 40 distinguished scholars from four continents in a tribute to our former publisher, Dr. Sadanand Singh, who had recently died, with all royalties going to the Sadanand Singh Foundation in San Diego. In his essay on "Defense Mechanisms and Coping Styles in Aphasia," Professor Tanner examined the role defense mechanisms and coping styles play in the psychological adjustment to aphasia. Nonverbal coping styles and defense mechanisms, such as denial, displacement, and projection, remain available, whereas those requiring language, such as rationalization, intellectualization, and humor, are partially or completely compromised.

Chapter previews and summaries in the book, as well as case reports and clinical illustrations, are useful pedagogical strategies to facilitate learning of complex material. Professor Tanner also includes his "Aphasic Patient's Bill of Rights." He leads us through the psychological minefields facing the person "wearing" aphasia (he stresses that the disorder is different from the individual), including the desolation of aphasia, the trauma of aphasia, the psychology of aphasia and the brain, the psychology of aphasia and the efficacy of therapy, major psychological issues in aphasia, and aphasia and quality of life, all in the first chapter.

Chapter 2 begins by examining the roles that different types of brain damage play in the psychology of aphasia and their predisposing effects for certain psychological reactions and disorders in patients with neurogenic communication disorders. These include perseveration and echolalia, emotional lability (I prefer the term "emotional incontinence," having experienced it), catastrophic reactions, organic depression-anxiety disorder, denial of impairment (anosognosia), visual neglect, euphoria, and maladaptive behavior.

In Chapter 3, Professor Tanner expands the themes of his translational speech-language pathology essay, with a more in-depth treatise on defense mechanisms and coping styles in aphasia. Included are external threats resulting in avoidance, ego restriction, escape, and autistic fantasy; as well as internal threats resulting in denial and repression. Other defense mechanisms and coping styles include psychological regression; passive aggression; reaction formation; displacement and projection; altruism, sublimation, and substitution; dissociation; inner speech; rationalization and intellectualization; suppression; undoing; and humor.

Chapter 4 deals with grief. Aphasia causes unwanted changes, with losses that may be tangible and/or symbolic. These include loss of relationships with important persons in the life of the patient, loss of some aspect of the patient's self, and loss of valued external objects. Professor Tanner discusses the importance of addressing and accepting unwanted changes, following Kübler-Ross' model of the grief response that relates to death and dying. He includes factors that affect the normal grieving process and those that can be influenced by the clinician or health care professional. Factors to avoid include rewarding denial, contributing to frustration, providing secondary gains, and interrupting private grief. He also recommends against using heavily sedating drugs, but is for permitting the patient control, providing the patient with perspective, and acknowledging the reality of the loss.

The Psychology of Aphasia: A Practical Guide for Health Care Professionals will be useful to the aphasia rehabilitation team of speech-language pathologists, psychologists, physical and occupational therapists, social workers, physicians and nurses, as well as family members and home health aides. I commend it to you all.

Robert Goldfarb, PhD, ASHA Fellow
Professor of Communication Sciences and Disorders
Adelphi University
Garden City, NY

REFERENCES

Goldfarb, R. (2015). An aphasiologist has a stroke. *Aphasiology*, DOI: 10.1080/02687038.2015.1092702

Goldfarb, R. (2016). An aphasiologist has a stroke. TEDx talk, available at https://www.youtube.com/watch?v=LLhXxBC9xYk

Tanner, D. C. (2012. Defense mechanisms and coping styles in aphasia In R. Goldfarb (Ed.), *Translation speech-language pathology and audiology: Essays in honor of Dr. Sadanand Singh* (pp. 301-306). San Diego: Plural.

INTRODUCTION

"But it must be said from the outset that a disease is never a mere loss or excess–that there is always a reaction, on the part of the affected organism or individual, to restore, to replace, to compensate for and to preserve its identity, however strange the means may be."

Oliver Sacks

Understanding the Psychology of Aphasia

Early in my education and throughout my 40+ year career, I have studied the psychological challenges and coping strategies of people with aphasia. As a scientist and professor, I have actively studied the psychology of aphasia and related disorders, and as a clinician through my company, Tanner Rehabilitation Services, Inc., evaluated and treated thousands of patients with neuropathologies of speech and language. With this book, I provide the reader with the culmination of my efforts to understand the major psychological aspects of this complex communication disorder. I have concluded that brain damage predisposes many people with aphasia to a variety of psychological reactions. These psychological reactions are precipitated by stress and loss, and perpetuated by impaired verbal defense mechanisms and coping styles.

Psychology of Aphasia: Brain Damage

I have served as an expert witness in many legal cases related to communication sciences and disorders. Most of them were medical malpractice cases, but some concerned speaker profiling and other forensic aspects of speech and hearing. I have written several books and journal articles on this subject including *The Medical-legal and Forensic Aspects of Communication Disorders*, *Voice Prints*, and *Speaker Profiling* (Lawyers & Judges Publishing). During my research for these cases, journal articles, and books, I became increasingly aware of the dramatic effects some brain injuries have on human behavior and can involve suicide, unprovoked aggression, denial, anxiety, depression, euphoria, criminal sexual acts, and a host of other aberrant actions and reactions. There is no question that brain injuries predispose some people to psychological actions and reactions, but the question remains why some people engage in them and others do not. While there is much research being conducted on psycho-organic aspects of the psychology of aphasia, little is known about patient-specific neurological factors.

Psychology of Aphasia: Impaired Verbal Defense Mechanisms

In 2012, I was invited to write an essay in the book: *Translational Speech-Language Pathology and Audiology: Essays in Honor of Dr. Sadanand Singh* (Plural Publishing). This was a professional honor for me because Dr. Sadanand Singh was a premier speech and hearing scientist and a man for whom I had the greatest respect. Consequently, I wrote "Defense Mechanisms and Coping Styles in Aphasia," which provided me with a large forum to dispense my current theories about the role impaired verbal defense mechanisms and coping styles play in the adjustment to aphasia. I have presented professional workshops and written about defense mechanisms and coping styles in aphasia in several of my books, and in the 2003 peer-reviewed *Journal of Allied Health* article entitled: "Eclectic Perspectives on the Psychology of Aphasia." Impaired verbal defense mechanisms and coping styles, seen particularly in global aphasia, is the second factor playing a major role in patients' adjustment to the loss of language. As you will read in this book, I explore the role compromised or lost abilities to engage in verbal defense mechanisms and coping styles have on a patient such as rationalization, intellectualization, humor, and undoing. The inability to use language to adjust to aphasia often leaves only nonverbal and perceptual defenses some of which are immature, radical, neurotic, and desperate attempts to cope with this potentially devastating disorder.

Psychology of Aphasia: Loss and Grief

I minored in psychiatry at Michigan State University where I received my doctorate in audiology and speech sciences. I was fortunate to have studied under Dr. John Schneider, who introduced me to the concepts of loss and grief after he had studied a new approach to coping with death and dying proposed by the renowned psychiatrist, Dr. Elisabeth Kübler-Ross, with the publication of her best-selling book: *On Death and Dying*. As a result of that educational experience, in 1980, I published "Loss and Grief: Implications for the Speech-Language Pathologist and Audiologist." It was the first cover article to appear in the *Journal of the American Speech-Language-Hearing Association* (ASHA). Over the next four decades, I built on Dr. Kübler-Ross' concepts of loss and grief and applied them to people with aphasia. In 1988, I and Dr. Dean Gerstenberger, a psychiatrist with whom I did a sabbatical, published an invited paper in the international, interdisciplinary journal *Aphasiology* entitled: "The Grief Response in Neuropathologies of Speech and Language." In 1996, the article was reprinted in the book: *Forums in Clinical Aphasiology* (Whurr Publishing). During the subsequent years, I published articles, books, and pamphlets about loss and grief emphasizing their relevance to people with aphasia. I also presented workshops on the topic at conventions of the American Speech-Language-Hearing Association.

A Practical Guide for Health Care Professionals

There is no shortage of academic books addressing the psychology of people with disabilities. Unfortunately, for practicing clinicians, these treatises often do not bridge the gap between "theoretical" and "practical" issues in treating actual patients. Too often, these books deal with abstractions, focus on the theoretical, and offer precious little guidance in dealing with actual patients. In the world of aphasia, what is written about the psychology of aphasia is often relegated to a chapter at the end of a book, and seemingly included only as an afterthought. More often than not, these books neglect the topic altogether.

The Psychology of Aphasia: A Practical Guide for Health Care Professionals is designed to provide the reader with a sound foundation of scientific information about the topic. There are current and historical scientific references to the psychology of aphasia spanning many decades. What is most important, the discussion of each major concept of the psychology of aphasia includes case studies, illustrations, and examples. These case studies, illustrations, and examples are written in accessible language and provide practical applications of the concepts. Some of them are actual case studies that come from my clinical experiences, and of course, names and other identifying information have been changed to protect the privacy of the people and institutions. Some case studies are brief synopses from my books: *Case Studies in Communication Sciences and Disorders*, 2nd edition (Slack Incorporated) and *The Family Guide to Surviving Stroke and Communication Disorders*, 2nd edition (Jones and Bartlett Publishers). Other case studies are drawn from reports from my colleagues, employees, and associates. Some are hypothetical examples and illustrations of the topics where I discuss the logical patient-specific applications. There is one poem, "The Silent Tongue," written by a registered nurse and award-winning poet after her sister acquired aphasia. These case studies, illustrations, and examples bridge the gap between the theories of the psychology of aphasia and application of them to specific patients.

As noted above, this book is the culmination of my decades-long study of the psychology of aphasia. Consequently, I draw from my published journal articles, scientific papers, and books on the subject. Specific and detailed information is taken from my books, *Exploring the Psychology, Diagnosis, and Treatment of Neurogenic Communication Disorders* and the *Psychology of Neurogenic Communication Disorders: A Primer for Health Care Professionals* both published or republished by iUniverse. The basis for the neuroanatomy and physiology discussions of the psycho-organic aspects of this book comes from *Anatomy and Physiology of Speech and Swallowing* (Kendall Hunt), and *Anatomy and Physiology Study Guide for Speech and Hearing* (Plural) coauthored by my colleagues Dr. William Culbertson and Dr. Stephanie Christensen. A journal article I wrote plays a prominent role in the information on receptive aphasia. "Redefining Wernicke's Area: Receptive Language and Discourse Semantics," published in the *Journal of Allied Health*, provides the basis for the discussion of persistent denial, projection, and jargon in Wernicke's aphasia.

The Psychology of Aphasia: Inductive and Deductive Logic

In this book, I base many of the concepts in the psychology of aphasia on scientific research. Science is based on inductive logic, or the "bottom up approach." In the scientific method, general conclusions are drawn from specific observations. Unfortunately, there is not enough scientific evidenced-based research to go around, not only for aphasia in general, but particularly its psychology.

To understand the scope and tone of this practical book, the reader will find elucidative, "Logical Alternatives to Aphasia Therapy When Evidence-Based Research Is Lacking," published and available as a tutorial in the *Journal of Medical Speech-Language Pathology*. In the article, I, with Dr. John Sciacca, theorize the use of logical deductive reasoning as an alternative to evidence-based research when the latter is lacking. In our article, we discuss deductive logic and the use of "clinical syllogisms" in aphasia therapy. A syllogism is a logical argument using deductive reasoning. Below is a famous syllogism:

Major premise: All men are mortal.

Minor premise: Aristotle is a man.

Conclusion: Aristotle is mortal.

Through deductive logic, you can see Aristotle is mortal (destined to die), based on the major and minor premises and the logical conclusion that follows. In "Logical Alternatives to Aphasia Therapy When Evidence-Based Research is Lacking," we developed three clinical syllogisms addressing intuition, authority, and relative application. Similar deductive reasoning is used herein to posit the concepts, illustrations, and examples not directly supported by evidenced-based research in the psychology of aphasia.

The Psychology of Aphasia: A Practical Guide for Health Care Professionals is the culmination of my exploration into the complex disorder of aphasia and its psychology. Some of the information is the result of my research, speculation, logical reasoning, and theorizing, but much came from the work of scientists, clinicians, aphasiologists, and scholars who preceded me. I am grateful to these remarkable men and women, and as Isaac Newton said, "If I have seen further it is by standing on the shoulders of Giants."

Dennis C. Tanner, PhD

1

Aphasia and Related Disorders

"Aphasia is a language problem, not a speech problem."

Frederic L. Darley

CHAPTER PREVIEW

This chapter defines and describes the neurogenic communication disorders of aphasia, apraxia of speech, dysarthrias, and the language of reduced or impaired consciousness seen in some people with traumatic brain injuries. This chapter discusses the etiology of aphasia, the brain-mind leap, language and symbolism, and brain localization issues. Emphasized is the importance of all health care professionals to address the psychology of aphasia and related disorders in therapies and treatments. There is a general overview of the three major psychological issues in aphasia to be discussed in this book: the effects of brain injury, psychological defense mechanisms and coping styles, and the grief response. Quality-of-life issues are defined, including their critical domains, and emphasizing psychological issues, changes, and challenges for people with aphasia.

THE "BIG THREE NEUROGENIC" COMMUNICATION DISORDERS

The "Big Three" communication disorders resulting from injury to the brain and/or nervous system are aphasia, apraxia of speech, and the dysarthrias. While these disorders can occur alone, they are often seen together. They are further divided into those that impair the fabric of language (aphasia) and those that are primarily motor speech disorders (apraxia of speech and the dysarthrias). As will be discussed below, aphasia refers to absent or impaired language functions, apraxia of speech is the impaired ability to program and execute neuromotor commands, and the dysarthrias are a collection of paralytic and movement neuromuscular disorders.

Tanner, D.C.
The Psychology of Aphasia: A Practical Guide for Health Care Professionals
(pp 1-32). © 2017 Taylor & Francis Group.

THE DESOLATION OF APHASIA

Of the multitude of diseases, defects, disorders, and disabilities afflicting humans, few can be as devastating as aphasia. Fortunately, some aphasias are mild and simply inconveniences; they have little effect on the patient's quality-of-life. Many of these aphasic symptoms resolve on their own, and they are insubstantial impairments to the ability to communicate. They do not substantially interfere with day-to-day family, work, and social activities. The communication disorders arising from these minor, and often temporary, disorders are nuisances and not life-altering barriers to quality living. Of course, there are individual differences in the way people deal with medical adversity. What is only minor and inconvenient to one person may be devastating to another. Nevertheless, as a rule, most people deal appropriately and proportionally with medical hardship, and these minor and often temporary aphasias are minimally disruptive to his or her overall quality-of-life.

Unfortunately, minor and temporary aphasias are rare. Most aphasias are substantial in severity and chronic, if not permanent. They often come on suddenly. For example, in stroke-related aphasias, there is little or no time for the patient to prepare for the medical emergency, and nearly instantaneously, he or she loses some or all of the ability to communicate. Other aphasias develop slowly, such as primary progressive aphasia, and those resulting from progressive degenerative diseases. Language impairments and abnormalities are sometimes the frightening initial symptoms of Alzheimer's disease and other dementias, and they can foretell the wasting of mental functions to follow. Initially, the symptoms may be barely noticeable, but overtime they can render the person completely unable to communicate with others. Aphasias caused by traumatic brain injuries occur violently, and they are often associated with major behavioral, cognitive, and emotional changes. Traumatic brain injuries are frequently associated with reduced or impaired consciousness.

Case Studies, Illustrations, and Examples: The Trauma of Aphasia

Your eyes slowly open. As the fluorescent light from the room gradually penetrates your brain, you feel a crisp sheet covering your body, and see a multitude of beeping, buzzing and dripping machines, clearly hospital in origin. The sterile white ceiling stares back at you, coldly indifferent to your plight. In an adjacent room, you hear doctors and nurses talking, conferring, ordering, and prescribing. Their words seem foreign and strange. In a blur of confusion, you fight to remember what brought you to this room. You have a vague recollection of a fall to the floor. You have other blurred images of an ambulance, gurney, blood pressure cuff, and flashing lights. You can feel sensors patched to your chest and arm, and a prickly needle penetrating a vein. You try to move your right arm, but it is to no avail. Your right arm muscles appear to be oblivious to your commands. To help them, you enlist the services of your left arm, but movement is abruptly restricted by a tightly tied restraint. You try to roll over to ease the back pain, but that too is futile. Your right leg will not move, clearly it is in cahoots with your stubborn right arm. Your mouth is as dry as a dust storm, and you feel a cloud of fear engulf you. You sense danger and succumb to an all-encompassing feeling of impending doom. Sweat appears on your brow and your stomach knots. Something terrible has happened and you know you must escape this danger. But physical escape is not an option. The path to safety is blocked by paralysis and restraints. You try and try again to escape this danger, but finally give-up and close your eyes. A woman in a white uniform utters a string of words you are incapable of understanding. You slip into the sanctuary of sleep as the nurse's word, "agitated," echoes in your mind.

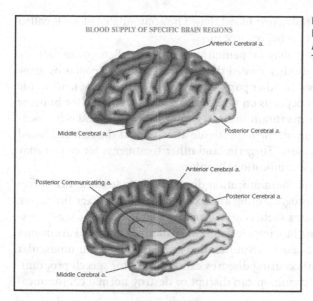

BLOOD SUPPLY OF SPECIFIC BRAIN REGIONS

Anterior Cerebral a.

Middle Cerebral a.   Posterior Cerebral a.

Anterior Cerebral a.

Posterior Communicating a.

Posterior Cerebral a.

Middle Cerebral a.

Figure 1-1. Blood supply to specific regions of the brain. (Reprinted with permission from Gutman, S. A. [2017.] *Quick Reference Neuroscience*, [3rd ed.]. Thorofare, NJ: SLACK Incorporated.)

ETIOLOGY OF APHASIA AND RELATED DISORDERS

Damage to the brain and nervous system can cause aphasia and other related neurogenic communication disorders. There are myriad medical events capable of causing neurogenic communication disorders, but the primary ones are strokes, tumors, cancer, diseases of the brain and nervous system, and traumatic brain injuries.

Strokes are a leading cause of death in the United States, and are the most common cause of neurogenic communication disorders. Strokes deprive the brain of blood, and when it is deprived for several minutes, neural tissue dies. There are two categories of vascular disturbances resulting in neurogenic communication disorders: occlusive and hemorrhagic.

An occlusive vascular accident is the result of the blockage of an artery. A blood clot or other obstruction can cause the blockage. It can also be caused by gradual decrease in the opening of blood vessels. When the blockage originates in the brain, it is called a cerebral thrombosis. "Most strokes are a thrombosis, which occurs from accumulation of atherosclerotic platelet and fatty plaque on the vessel wall at the site of occlusion" (Davis, 2007, p. 20). A cerebral embolus is a blockage originating elsewhere in the body, and eventually lodging in the brain. Two or more emboli are called a "shower of emboli." How much brain damage resulting from the occlusion is dependent upon the completeness of the blockage, and the size of the area of the brain that was deprived of blood. When a small area of the brain is deprived of blood, there is generally less damage to communicative functions than if the damaged area is large. However, some small focalized areas of brain damage may cause major neurogenic communication disorders. Figure 1-1 shows the blood supply to specific regions of the brain.

A transient ischemic attack (TIA) is sometimes referred to as a ministroke. It is a temporary disruption of blood flow in the brain and often foretells an impending stroke. During a transient ischemic attack, the patient may have neurogenic communication disorders typical of a stroke, which remit after the TIA is over. A stroke-in-evolution is an ongoing disruption in blood flow to the brain.

A hemorrhagic stroke is caused by a blow-out of a blood vessel, and is usually associated with high blood pressure or brain trauma. A ruptured aneurysm causes some hemorrhages. An aneurysm is a weakening of the arterial wall and a ballooning of an artery. When a blood vessel hemorrhages, the area served by the vessel is deprived of blood and there is spilling of it elsewhere, often causing increased pressure in the brain and restricting blood flow. The accumulated blood is called a hematoma and may have to be evacuated by a neurosurgeon.

A tumor is also called a neoplasm and it may be benign or malignant. Benign tumors are space-occupying and can cause aphasia and other related disorders. Malignant neoplasms grow uncontrolled and can metastasize and spread to other parts of the body. The types of neurogenic communication disorders caused by tumors depends on their severity and location in the brain or nervous system. Malignant cerebral neoplasms (brain tumors) can cause aphasia and other neurogenic communication disorders depending on the brain tissue affected and the reduced blood circulation caused by increased cranial pressure. Surgeries and other treatments for cancer may also damage tissue and cause neurogenic communication disorders.

Other diseases that can cause neurogenic communication disorders include those that affect neuromuscular functioning, motor speech programming and execution, and language functions. For example, progressive degenerative diseases such as amyotrophic lateral sclerosis (ALS), muscular dystrophy (MD), and multiple sclerosis (MS) impair neuromuscular functioning. Parkinson's disease (PD), caused by the deficiency of the neurotransmitter dopamine, disrupts neuromuscular functioning. Alzheimer's and other dementia causing diseases can affect motor speech programming and execution. Any disease affecting cognition can disrupt or destroy normal communication functions.

There are two types of traumatic head injuries: closed and open. A closed head injury is caused by a blunt force trauma to the head resulting in acceleration and deceleration of the brain. When this occurs, neurons and other tissue within the brain are torn. In an open head injury, a projectile or missile penetrates the skull and brain. Common projectiles include bullets fired from guns and shrapnel. Both open and closed head traumas can cause focalized and diffuse brain injuries and hemorrhages. Traumatic brain injury can minimally or completely disrupt language, motor speech programming and execution, and neuromuscular functioning. The site, extent, and nature of the traumatic brain injury determines the symptoms presented by the patient. Since traumatic brain injuries are so variable, there are three diagnostic factors related to the etiology of neurogenic communication disorders.

First, a small percentage of people with traumatic brain injuries primarily have focalized damage to the major speech and language centers of the brain. Since there is focalized damage, these patients have neurogenic communication disorders typically seen in many stroke patients. Second, some patients have traumatically induced brain and/or nervous system damage, but the major speech and language centers are spared. Although these patients may have problems communicating, the fabric of language and the motor speech functions remain intact. These patients primarily present with the "language of confusion." They may have problems with arousal, orientation, behavior, judgment, retrograde and anterograde amnesias, and posttraumatic psychosis. Third, patients with traumatic brain injuries, particularly those with severe injuries, often have aphasia, apraxia of speech, and the dysarthrias compounded by arousal, orientation, behavior, judgment, retrograde and anterograde amnesias, and posttraumatic psychosis. Pachaiska, Jastrzebowska, Gryglicka, Mirska, and Macqueen (2015) concluded that aphasia is not the only, or even the most important, cause of communication disorders in patients with traumatic brain injuries. Table 1-1 shows the cognitive and behavioral disorders in patients with the "language of confusion." Table 1-2 illustrates the three primary variations of neurogenic communication disorders associated with traumatic brain injury.

TABLE 1-1
COGNITIVE AND BEHAVIORAL DISORDERS
IN THE LANGUAGE OF CONFUSION

FUNCTION	DISORDER	DESCRIPTION
Awareness	Coma, stupor, delirium, clouding of consciousness	Absent or reduced awareness of self and environment
Reality Testing	Posttraumatic psychosis	Break with one or more aspects of reality: hallucinations and delusions
Memory	Retrograde and anterograde amnesia	Memory loss of events before and/or after the TBI, problems learning
Orientation	Disorientation to time, place, person, and/or situation (predicament)	Confusion about time events and/or the passage of time, people (including self), place, and the reason for hospitalization

TABLE 1-2
PRIMARY VARIATIONS OF NEUROGENIC COMMUNICATION DISORDERS

FOCALIZED TRAUMATIC BRAIN INJURY AFFECTING THE MAJOR SPEECH LANGUAGE CENTERS/TRACTS	TRAUMATIC BRAIN INJURY NOT AFFECTING THE MAJOR SPEECH AND LANGUAGE CENTERS/TRACTS	DIFFUSE BRAIN INJURY ALSO AFFECTING THE MAJOR SPEECH AND LANGUAGE CENTERS/TRACTS
Classic Aphasia Classic Apraxia of Speech Classic Dysarthria	Impaired or Reduced Consciousness Affecting Mental Executive Functions, Orientation, and Memory	Aphasia, Apraxia of Speech, and the Dysarthrias Compounded and Complicated by Reduced or Impaired Consciousness

DEFINING APHASIA AND RELATED DISORDERS

Before discussing the psychology of aphasia, it is necessary to define the disorder and to distinguish it from other neurogenic communication disorders. This is particularly important when discussing the psychology of aphasia because people with aphasia have psychological issues, changes, and challenges different from those individuals with apraxia of speech and the dysarthrias. In addition, due to the communication disorder, traditional "talking cures" are impractical and oftentimes ineffective, ineffectual, or even useless. Counseling and psychotherapy may actually exacerbate psychological issues, changes, and challenges in a person with aphasia because of the increased frustration associated with impaired communication. When discussing psychological aspects of aphasia, it is important to recognize that aphasia is not a speech pathology; it is a language disturbance. It affects, more or less, all modalities, or avenues, of language expression and

Figure 1-2. Modalities of language.

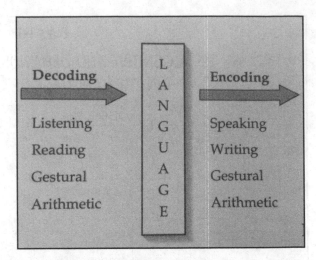

Figure 1-3. Aphasia cuts across all modalities of communication

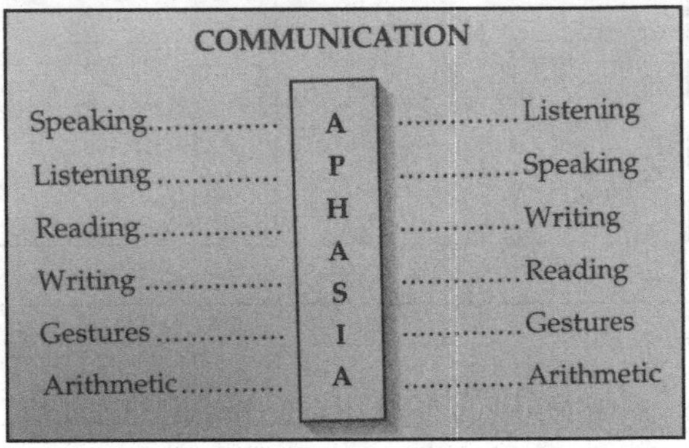

reception (Figure 1-2). The expressive modalities of language affected by aphasia include speaking, writing, mathematic expression, and the use of complex gestures for communication purposes. The receptive modalities of language are auditory comprehension, reading, mathematical understanding, and comprehension of complex gestures. Figure 1-3 illustrates that aphasia cuts across all modalities or avenues of communication.

Neurogenic communication disorders are a general category of disorders arising from damage to the brain and nervous system. They encompass aphasia, motor speech disorders (apraxia of speech and the dysarthrias), the speech pathologies, reduced or impaired consciousness, and language impairments seen in traumatic brain injury. The following definitions are the basis for the discussions of the psychology of aphasia to follow:

Aphasia: An acquired loss or disruption of language due to damage to the major speech and language centers of the brain; the multimodality inability or impaired ability to encode, decode, and manipulate symbols for the purposes of verbal thought and/or communication.

Apraxia of Speech (verbal apraxia): The inability or impaired ability to conceptualize, program, and execute voluntary neuromuscular speech movements.

Dysarthrias: A general category of neuromuscular disorders resulting from damage to the brain and nervous system. The dysarthrias affect the timing, strength, range-of-motion, speed, and/or appropriateness of motor speech movements. They affect one or more of the five motor speech processes of respiration, phonation, articulation, resonance, and prosody.

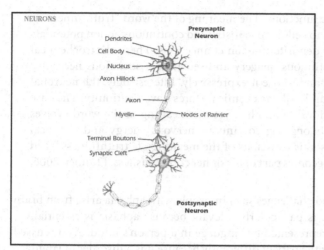

Figure 1-4. The neuron propagates ionic changes, action potentials, which travel from dendrites to axons. (Reprinted with permission from Gutman, S. A. [2017.] *Quick Reference Neuroscience*, [3rd ed.]. Thorofare, NJ: SLACK Incorporated.)

Language of Reduced or Impaired Consciousness: Language reflecting reduced or impaired consciousness is often associated with memory impairments, disorientation, and disordered mental executive functions. It is sometimes referred to as the "language of confusion" and is typically seen in patients with traumatic brain injury.

There are four important distinctions in the definition of aphasia. First, aphasia is a multimodality communication disorder. Although a particular patient may present with predominantly expressive or predominantly receptive symptoms, aphasia, more or less, cuts across all modalities of language. Second, there are degrees of aphasia and the symptoms naturally evolve in type and severity. Third, predominantly expressive aphasia primarily disrupts encoding of language and predominantly receptive aphasia is primarily a disorder of language decoding. Fourth, aphasia as a language disorder, affects the psychological processing of verbal symbols.

THE BRAIN-MIND LEAP

An issue challenging neuroscientists, theologians, and philosophers for centuries is the so-called "brain-mind leap." The brain-mind leap is the scientific and philosophical process of projecting the neurological activity in the brain and nervous system to what occurs in a person's mind. At the brain level, consciousness, thought, speech, and language are electrochemical impulses traveling along nerve axons and dendrites to synaptic junctions. Neurological impulses are actions of nerve fibers and electrical charges traveling from neuron to neuron and involving several chemical reactions at the synaptic level. The neuron propagates ionic changes, action potentials, which travel from dendrites to axons (Figure 1-4). All consciousness, thought, speech, and language are the result of activities and changes in brain chemistry and these neuronal connections. The scientific, religious, and philosophical issues in the brain-mind leap are how these chemical and neuronal activities in a person's brain become consciousness, thought, speech, and language. According to Davis (2007), aphasiology was born with a neurological orientation more than one hundred years ago, whereas a scientific approach to the mind emerged only in the 1970s. Davis (2007, p. 9) goes on to remark: "The brain and the mind are not usually treated as alternative versions of the truth."

There is no better example of the inherent difficulties and challenges involved in the brain-mind leap than in language functioning, and particularly abstract semantics.

The magnitude of the brain-mind leap can be demonstrated by addressing semantic representations in the brain. Neurologically, the meaning of the word "truthfulness," for example, can be found in the atomic particles in neurons, and the chemical interactions of neurotransmitters at their synaptic junctions. The meaning of the word "truthfulness" is likely a composite of these changes to cellular chemistry and continuous action potentials in thousands of neurons and their dendrite-to-axon connections. These electrochemical reactions somehow create the continuous imagery and semantic associations necessary to sense the meaning of the word and to use it expressively. Interestingly, the neuronal impulses, their action potentials, and cellular chemical stores have continuity. They are consistent from one semantic retrieval to another, yet the meaning of the word evolves with life experience. Through this ongoing continuous nervous energy and chemical changes at the cellular level, a person is conscious of the meaning of "truthfulness," and in fact, the semantics of the word becomes part of his or her consciousness. (Tanner, 2006, pp. 162-163)

The psychological issues, changes, and challenges seen in people with aphasia arise from brain damage, and the brain-mind leap issue is particularly relevant because aphasia is essentially a disorder of symbolism where reality is represented by language in a person's mind. As discussed below, aphasia itself is conceptualized by the patient differently because it is a disorder of language and symbolism.

LANGUAGE AND SYMBOLISM

To fully understand the psychology of aphasia, it is necessary to review the nature of language and symbolism. Language is symbolic, and aphasia is a symbolic neurogenic communication disorder. Non-symbolic neurogenic communication disorders include apraxia of speech and the dysarthrias which often occur with aphasia. A "symbol" is an entity that represents something else. In language, the symbol can be graphic, verbal, or gestural, and that to which it refers is the "referent." Symbols are abstractions; they are generalizations from specific aspects of reality. Lev Vygotsky (1896-1934), a Russian linguist, observed that a word refers to a class of objects rather than a single one, thus generalizing reality differently than an image or other sensation (Vygotsky, 1962).

Semantics, the substance of language, lies in the symbol-referent relationship and is the foundation to all meaning in language. The symbol-referent relationship is dynamic because language symbols and their meanings change over time. In fact, the meaning of a language symbol changes every time it is used because of the passage of time and the ever-changing nature of reality. Language symbols are also arbitrary; they are randomly created and used by a language community. There are no physical laws or mental requirements that a series of phonemes (sounds) or graphemes (letters) represent a particular entity. Each language community establishes an arbitrary set of symbols to represent reality.

Aphasia affects linguistic performance and competence. Linguistic performance is the use of language in everyday conversation; it is the person's actual use of language. Linguistic competence, possessed by native users of a language, is the knowledge of the language codes. Grammar is a general term for the rules of the form and usage of a language. Contrary to the arbitrary nature of semantics, grammar gives stability, predictability, form, and order to language. According to Campbell (1982, p. 165), "Grammar which is part of [language] competence, acts as a filter screening out errors and incorrect arrangements of words, showing a speaker which sentence forms are admissible, and whether they are connected with certain other sentence forms by rules of transformation."

Expressive language involves encoding or synthesizing thoughts into a linguistic code. This is the process of synthesizing sensory information, perceptions of reality, and thought into linguistic units: phonology, syntax, semantics, and pragmatics. Phonology is the study of the speech sounds of a language and the way they are combined into syllables and words. Syntax is the linguistic rules for arranging units of meaning into connected utterances. As discussed above, semantics is the meaning of morphemes (the smallest units of meaning), words, phrases, and discourse. Expressive language also involves pragmatics and the application of meaning to a particular communicative circumstance or context. Receptive language is the decoding or analyzing of these linguistic units.

There are six primary modalities or avenues of communicative expression and reception. Expressively, communicators speak, write, or express themselves with gestures. Receptively, communicators understand what is spoken, read, and can decipher these expressive gestures. Encoding of thoughts spoken involves speech sound production. Writing is creating meaning with graphemes, and gesturing uses meaningful physical movements to transmit information. Decoding speech is the process of analyzing auditory signals. Reading is the deciphering of graphemes into meaningful linguistic units. An important difference between reading and writing and other modalities affected by aphasia is that both reading and writing must be taught. While most humans are born with the ability to use and understand the other modalities of communication, a person must be taught to read and write–to understand and give meaning to written symbols. Gestural comprehension is the attachment of meaning to gestured physical movements during communication. Mathematics is also a language with expressive and receptive modalities. Mathematics uses conventional language symbols and unique or conventional ones with different or expanded meanings, too.

In adults, language and abstract thought are fundamentally connected. In young children, language primarily represents thought. Young children are on a concrete level, and words and other utterances reflect what is occurring in their minds. In adults, language not only reflects concrete thought, but it is fundamental to abstract thinking primarily because adults use internal monologues or inner speech in cognition. Abstract linguistic constructs, such as verbally pondering whether it is ethical to engage in a particular behavior, and processing individual words such as "truthfulness," "inevitable," and "friendship," are cognitive processes that do not derive themselves from tangible objective referents. However, even tangible words and concepts involve abstraction. Sternberg and Ben-Zeev (2001, p. 202) note that even when a person is thinking about the tangible word "chair," he or she also conjures: 1) all of the instances of chairs in existence anywhere, 2) instances of chairs that exist only in the imagination, 3) all the characteristics of chairs, 4) all the things that may be done with chairs and, 5) all the other concepts linked to chairs (e.g., things you put on a chair or places where you may find chairs). These abstractions can be viewed as cognitively processing "chairness."

Language, and its inherent symbolism, is fundamental in dealing with the unwanted changes brought about by aphasia. Psychologically, aphasia is a triple-edged sword. It is the cause of a myriad of changes, impairments, and disabilities. Due to the symbolic nature of aphasia, it affects the very conceptualization of the disorder and the person's coping and adjustment abilities. The breakdown in communication between the patient and his or her loved ones complicates the psychological issues, changes, and challenges and further isolates those with aphasia. In the poem below, an award-winning poet captures the isolation and discontentment experienced by her aphasic sister.

Case Studies, Illustrations, and Examples: "The Silent Tongue"

The Silent Tongue (aphasia)

The words you do not hear the tears you cannot see

Are hidden within my nucleus, this is my new identity

I am alike dry earth, shriveled and worn

With no nurturing to the soul

And I am quite helpless, in my world no longer whole.

So bear with me and try to creep inside this silent tent

My ills have bereaved my spirit

My soul is discontent.

Please do not look at me … as if I am not here

Please do not speak to me … as if I cannot hear

Although I can't express myself with this muted speech of mine

My needs are very important it's difficult to define.

Please be polite and patient … maintain my dignity

My mind is tired and weary with this disability

I sit in silence in my room I cannot say "Good Morning Sun"

The words are tangled in my mind

Like twisted branches on a vine.

Those who speak in silence have a fervor

We … Who talk so freely don't understand or know

Take a walk into a garden, see the flowers row on row

Their colors are bright, their life is sweet

And we hear words of passion in the silent way they speak.

Kathleen Gerety, RN

Atkinson, New Hampshire

Copyright 2017 by Dennis C. Tanner (Originally published in Tanner, D. (2003). *The Psychology of Neurogenic Communication Disorders: A Primer for Health Care Professionals*. Boston, MA: Allyn & Bacon)

PSYCHOLOGY OF APHASIA AND THE BRAIN

The thrust of early research into neurogenic communication disorders was to locate, or localize, areas of the brain responsible for specific speech and language functions. Review of early research into the psychology of aphasia and the brain provides a foundation for understanding the current theories and philosophies about this complicated disorder. This desire to localize functional speech and language areas of the brain, or "modules," continues today.

A strict localizationist philosophy of brain functioning is difficult to support. No single part of the brain functions completely independent from the others. For example, although there may be certain identifiable areas of the brain important in perceiving vowels and consonants, pointing to a mass of brain cells completely responsible, in every person, for interpreting a proverb or understanding the implications of a Robert Frost poem is absurd. As discussed previously, there also is the monumental task of identifying the neurochemical activities in the neurons and cells of the brain and projecting what happens in a particular person's mind. Given current technology and scientific advances, the brain-mind leap is insurmountably complex and compounded by extreme individual variation.

In the past, as today, not all scientists and clinicians in neurogenic communication disorders were swept up in the popular localization movement. An early critic of the theories of localization was Henry Head (1861-1940). Head was particularly critical of the researchers of the day who assumed that "pure" neurogenic speech and language disorders existed. Head believed it was unproductive to list speech and language functions, and to create a diagram showing the areas of the brain responsible for all of them. Head recognized that the brain operates holistically. In Head's 1926 classic textbook on aphasia, *Aphasia and Kindred Disorders of Speech*, he sarcastically referred to localizationists as "diagram makers."

Over time, "schools of thought" regarding aphasia and related disorders were formed. Perhaps it is because of the complexity of these disorders that many present-day scientists and clinicians adhere so rigidly to the doctrines of those philosophies. Those early schools of thought, and many others, make basic assumptions about the cognitive and psychological makeup of patients with neurogenic communication disorders.

The "association" school of thought assumes that aphasic disorders are disturbances in labeling ideas, objects, or events. Adherents to this school think that the basic intellectual capacity of the patient remains essentially intact. Associationists regard intellectual activity as a function of large areas of the brain working as a whole. What is most significant about the "association" school of thought is that it regards intelligence as located outside the region bounded by the language centers of the brain.

The "cognitive" school rejects the idea that thought and language are separate entities. Armand Trousseau (1801-1867) first challenged the idea that thought could be largely unimpaired in aphasia. Trousseau believed that intelligence always was "lamed" in aphasia. He challenged the belief that language simply expresses thought in adults. The cognitive school takes a more holistic approach to aphasia.

John Hughlings Jackson (1835-1911) was the first aphasiologist to systematically study the patient's "psyche." In this dimension of the study of aphasia and related disorders, Jackson was a pioneer. For the first time, patients suffering from aphasia were viewed in a comprehensive manner that did not include the artificial separation of thought, speech, language, and the patient's psyche. He proposed a unitary, psychological approach to brain functioning. Jackson fused thought, language and the individual's intent in communicating to the study of aphasia and related disorders.

Jackson also applied the concept of inner speech to the study of aphasia. He believed that all forms of speech were similar and that inner speech–internal monologues–occur with the same structure as other propositional utterances. In Jackson's, *On Affections of Speech from Diseases of the Brain*, he discussed the "proposition" as it relates to externalized and inner speech.

> To speak is not simply to utter words, it is to propositionise. A proposition is such a relation of words that it makes one new meaning; not by a mere addition of what we call the separate meanings of the several words; the terms of the proposition are modified by each other. Single words are meaningless, and so is any unrelated succession of words. The unit of speech is the proposition. A single word is, or is in effect, a proposition, if other words in relation are implied. (Jackson, 1878, p. 311)

Weisenburg and McBride (1935) were concerned with more than speech responses and neurology. They are credited with doing the first truly scientific study of aphasia. Unfortunately, their conclusions about the performance of aphasic subjects were questionable because of a flawed research design; their subjects were not neurologically stable at the time of testing. They observed that aphasia affects the patient's reactions to practical and social situations. Although they did not identify complex personality changes in their patients, they did view aphasia as a syndrome inclusive of attitudinal and emotional changes. Schuell, Jenkins, and Jimenez-Pabon (1964, p. 44) summarized their study as timeless: "Good clinical observations are never dated and in this respect this is a timeless study."

Holistic theories of aphasia were furthered by Kurt Goldstein (1878-1965). Goldstein is best known for postulating an "abstract-concrete imbalance" in aphasic patients' performance of reasoning tasks. Goldstein theorized that the aphasic patient has specific deficiencies in maintaining an "abstract attitude." This loss of abstract attitude is present, not only in language, but in nonverbal performance tasks such as sorting colors and classifying objects. The loss of the abstract attitude in aphasia reflects the power of language to engage in abstract thought.

Goldstein was influenced by gestalt psychology and consequently viewed aphasia from a broad theoretical perspective. Goldstein's gestalt psychology background provided a basis for his initial theories into the aphasic patient's ego. Goldstein viewed the aphasic patient as one suffering from a concrete attitude and bound to immediate experience.

Joseph Wepman (1962) discussed the effects of aphasia on the patient's ego and self-concept: "In every instance of brain damage there appears to be some degree of ego weakness and disruption of the self-concept" (p. 207). A patient with a weak or negative self-concept is likely to have distorted perceptions and seek to defend himself or herself. According to Wepman, the patient must reorganize his or her self-concept, and realistically assess his or her strengths and weaknesses. "The self-concept evolved must be in terms of the patient as he is, facing the reality of his condition and leaving the 'ghost of the past' that so often haunts him" (Wepman, 1962, p. 207). Wepman considered aphasia not only a language disorder, but a psychological impairment as well and affecting the patients' entire personality.

Wepman considered aphasia to be a regression in linguistic and cognitive functioning. According to the linguistic regression theory, the speechlessness of an infant corresponds to the most severe category of language disturbance: global aphasia. The stage of language development in which the child acquires vocabulary correlates with semantic aphasia. Syntactic aphasia roughly correlates with the grammatical acquisition stages of the child. He believed that the stages of recovery from aphasia should parallel these developmental stages. The unfortunate consequence of this flawed theory was to characterize people with aphasia as childlike and simple-minded.

The noted Soviet neuropsychologist A. R. Luria (1902-1977) took exception with the linguistic regression theory, and extended the argument to psychological reactions. He suggested that pathological states of the brain do not return the individual to stages of development he or she has previously passed, the effects of learning and experience are too strong. The patient's previous experiences cannot leave him or her unchanged, even after extensive brain damage. According to Luria, voluntary activity does not originate from "primordial" properties; the human experience is a process of transformation, which leaves the adult unique and psychologically different from the child.

Russell Brain (1895-1966) and Macdonald Critchley (1900-1997) are considered pioneers in the neurology of aphasia, and they appreciated the importance of the psychology of the patient. Brain (1965) concluded that aphasia is more than a neurological event; it must be considered on a psychological level. Critchley (1970) explored the use of inner symbols of the aphasic patient and postulated the existence of a grammar to internal monologues. The grammar of internal monologues gives structure and order to the silent thinking process.

Norman Geschwind (1926-1984) studied naming errors in aphasic patients and has been in the forefront in localizing language disturbances. Geschwind identified several types of aphasia including hysterical anomia (difficulty remembering words) occurring as a manifestation of hysteria or malingering. Hysterical anomia may be the only abnormality presented by the patient, or it may occur as one symptom of a more complicated hysterical syndrome.

John Sarno (1981) addressed the need for a logical way to address the psychology of aphasia, and suggested "ground rules" for a "science of emotions." Categorical separation of groups for study should include:

> Patients with unilateral stroke (with the lesion in the distribution of one vessel only), space-occupying tumors, invasive tumors, missile wounds, head trauma with focal

lesions (lacerations, loss of substance, intracerebral hemorrhage, peridural hemorrhage), head trauma without focal lesions and with coma. (Sarno, J., 1981, p. 481)

Although etiology can certainly affect the psychology of aphasia, separating them into these small subgroups too narrowly restricts them for theoretical utility.

Jon Eisenson (1907-2001) has been in the forefront of appreciating the psychological effects of aphasia. "We would consider it surprising if an individual who has incurred a cerebral insult and associated aphasic disturbances did not undergo consequent changes in personality" (Eisenson, 1984, p. 87). According to Eisenson, an impairment of language affects the manner in which the personality is manifest and there are disruptions in the capacity for planning. Those who make expected good recoveries are those who adjust to the brain damage, and those who do not reach their potential are hindered by their premorbid inclinations and ego involvement. Eisenson explained the role of ego involvement in the aphasic patient who does not make appreciable improvement with ordinary motivation: "Their inclination, their needs, their interpretations, rather than those of their cultural environment, become the dominant ones. Thus, verbal expressions have limited meanings and restricted significance" (Eisenson, 1984, p. 91).

Aphasia may be more accurately defined as a "disorder of a person" than a "disorder of language" (Sarno, M., 1991). A holistic approach is warranted for those patients with personality and emotional dysfunctions associated with aphasia. The diagnosis and treatment of aphasia are dynamic processes. The fact that these disorders evolve in type and severity overtime requires ongoing reevaluation not only of the speech and language symptoms, but also the important psychological aspects of them.

Leonard LaPointe (1997) proposed that aphasia and related disorders should be understood in the context of adapting to chronic illness. Adaptation and accommodation to chronic illness involves going from uncertainty, to regaining wellness through taking charge, setting goals, seeking closure, and attaining mastery over it. Of special importance in adapting to these serious illnesses are the support and encouragement provided by family and friends and all members of the rehabilitation team working together on psychiatric considerations (Baker and Tanner, 1990; Scott and Tanner, 1990).

More recent contemporary neuroscientists use advanced techniques for studying the brain, which has increased the rate of learning about its functions. These include computed tomography (CT), magnetic resonance imaging (MRI), single photon tomography (SPECT), positron emission tomography (PET), functional magnetic resonance imaging (fMRI), magnetoencephalography (MEG), near infrared spectroscopy (NIS), and others.

To no small part, the discipline of aphasiology was born from debate over localized versus holistic explanations of the functions in the brain. Rarely has the study of these disorders been free from controversy, and the psychology of them is no exception. As a result, the localization movement is not dead, but it has changed. There have been refinements in the armament of the academic war, but many issues remain stubbornly present. The nature of aphasia and related disorders is resistant to consensus because to know these neuropathologies of speech and language is to understand the essence of human thought.

PERCEPTION AND THE AGNOSIAS

To understand the psychology of aphasia, and to appreciate the complexity of language processing, it is important to distinguish sensory "perception" from language "association." Perception occurs with each of the five senses: vision, hearing, touch, taste, and smell. Sensation is the detection of environmental stimuli and involves sense organs such as the eye, skin, and ear. Perception, Latin from "percipere" or "to take in completely," is a higher neurological, mental, and psychological level of information processing than sensation. Perception allows awareness of what is sensed

Figure 1-5. Senses and corresponding agnosias.

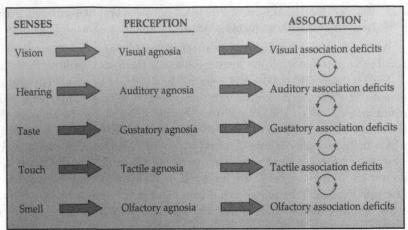

and is the first stage of attaching meaning to environmental stimuli. Perception is the process of attending to the "significant" and "important" sensory information, and the routing of it for higher cortical processing. Mentally, perception lies between sensory and associative cognitive functions.

In the late 1800s, Sigmund Freud first coined the term "agnosia" as a perceptual disorder. Benson and Ardila (1996) described agnosia as a percept without its meaning and a general lack of recognition. Jon Eisenson (1984, p. 10) considered agnosia a frequently occurring disorder in aphasia: "Such impairments of perception have serious implications for language if they involve auditory or visual modalities or, in the case of blind persons, the tactile modality." While aphasic disorders, to varying degrees, affect all modalities of communication, agnosias are usually limited to one modality. They are breakdowns in information processing occurring between the senses and associative functions of the cortex (Figure 1-5).

Classifying Aphasia

There are many classification systems of aphasia and each reflects a theory about the nature of this neurogenic communication disorder. This has led to controversy about the characteristics to which each aphasia diagnostic label refers, and led to a "chaos of classifications." Below is a discussion of the aphasia diagnostic terminology commonly used by neuroscientists, aphasiologists, physicians, speech-language pathologists, and other health care professionals involved in the evaluation and treatment of patients so affected. It includes neuroanatomical sites, fluency factors, anterior-posterior designations, and motor-sensory distinctions.

Table 1-3 shows three general classification categories, the assumed primary site of brain and central nervous system damage, and conventional terminology for specific aphasia diagnostic labels. The neuroanatomical reference sites of lesions are Broca's area, Wernicke's area, and/or the tracts of the brain leading to and from them.

In the early 1900s, Korbinian Brodmann (1868-1918), a German neurologist, created the brain mapping system that bears his name. He identified 52 functional sites of the brain based on their stained visual appearance. Later, some of the original sites were further subdivided to more clearly reflect their location and function. Broca's area is located in Brodmann area 44, which is the inferior frontal gyrus of the left cerebral hemisphere. Most authorities also include Brodmann area 45, the pars triangularis of the inferior frontal gyrus, as part of Broca's area. The left precentral gyrus is associated with apraxia of speech in acute aphasia (Itabashi, et al., 2015). Wernicke's area is located in Brodmann Areas 22, 41, and 42 in the superior part of the left temporal lobe which is also

TABLE 1-3 THREE GENERAL APHASIA CATEGORIES		
DAMAGE TO BROCA'S AND/OR ADJACENT AREAS/TRACTS OF THE BRAIN	**DAMAGE TO WERNICKE'S AND/OR ADJACENT AREAS/TRACTS OF THE BRAIN**	**DAMAGE TO BROCA'S, WERNICKE'S, AND/OR ADJACENT AREAS/TRACTS OF THE BRAIN**
Broca's aphasia	Wernicke's aphasia	Global aphasia
Predominantly expressive aphasia	Predominantly receptive aphasia	Severe expressive-receptive aphasia
Motor aphasia	Sensory aphasia	Dense aphasia
Nonfluent aphasia	Fluent jargon aphasia	Irreversible aphasia syndrome
Anterior aphasia	Posterior aphasia	Anterior-posterior, mixed aphasia

known as the superior temporal area and the primary auditory cortex. Some authorities extend the Wernicke's area into the parietal lobe including Brodmann area 39 and Brodmann area 40 and the angular and supramarginal sections, which are involved in reading and alexia. The diagnostic labels of "Broca's aphasia" and "Wernicke's aphasia" refer to damage to the above areas and/or the tracts leading to and from them. Figure 1-6 shows approximate sites of major speech and hearing landmarks of the brain. It should be noted that the so-called "speech and language centers" are not "centers" for expressive and receptive language, but "conduits" for language processing; especially in regard to language and discourse because the brain operates as a whole (Tanner, 2007). Fridriksson, Fillmore, Dazahou, and Rorden (2015) recently reported that chronic Broca's aphasia is caused by damage to Broca's and Wernicke's areas.

Some authorities on aphasia use the motor-sensory aphasia distinction. For the purposes of the discussion of the psychology of aphasia, "motor aphasia" is an oxymoron. Since "pure" aphasia is a language disorder and not a speech pathology, motor aphasia is a contradiction in diagnostic terms. Motor aphasia, an expressive disorder, results from damage to Broca's area and/or adjacent areas and tracts of the brain. The reference of "motor" refers to the impairment of programming seen in apraxia of speech which often accompanies language encoding disorders. "Sensory aphasia," a receptive disorder, results from damage to Wernicke's area and/or adjacent areas and tracts of the brain. The concept of sensory aphasia is also misleading because it suggests the problems with decoding language is a result of a sensory dysfunction such as a hearing loss. Extensive damage to both areas is sometimes called "global aphasia" or "dense aphasia" referring to a large mass of brain and central nervous system damage.

In the "nonfluent-fluent" aphasia diagnostic terminology in Table 1-3, the patient's speech and language fluency distinguishes expressive and receptive impairments. Non-fluent aphasia, an expressive aphasia, includes decreased output, effort and struggle to produce speech, decreased phrase length, and prosodic disturbances. Motor speech disorders are often present in non-fluent aphasia. Fluent aphasia, a receptive aphasia, is associated with reduced auditory and reading comprehension, and the expressive component is sometimes referred to as fluent jargon aphasia. Fluent aphasia speakers produce speech with little effort and struggle, and with normal prosody, but the output often is semantically inappropriate or meaningless. The structure of fluent aphasia appears normal, but the content is without meaning. "Thus, although they speak at a quite normal speaking rate, sounds shift and words blend in their speech. Sometimes whole utterances consist

Figure 1-6. Approximate boundaries of expressive and receptive speech and language centers.

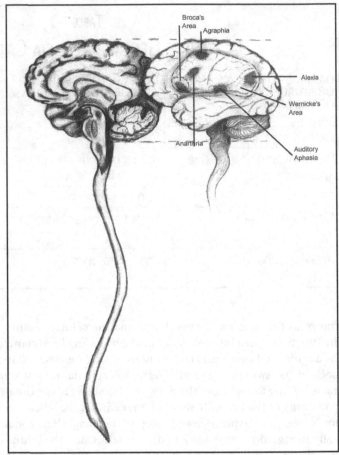

of neologisms, nonexisting words that sound like but are not words of the speaker's language" (Laakso, 2003, p. 163). Severe damage to the important speech and language centers of the brain, such as is seen in global aphasia, is considered irreversible.

In the anterior and posterior aphasia distinction, the dividing neuroanatomical line is the fissure of Rolando, also called the central sulcus or central fissure. The fissure of Rolando separates the frontal and parietal lobes. Anterior aphasia is non-fluent and agrammatic. Patients with anterior aphasia have problems writing, using expressive gestures, and repeating. Posterior aphasia is fluent albeit meaningless. Patients with posterior aphasia have problems reading and understanding the speech and complicated gestures of others. Damage to both regions is mixed or anterior-posterior aphasia.

LANGUAGE ENCODING DISORDERS

Language encoding is formulating and transforming cognitive information into an expressive linguistic code. It is the process by which humans express thoughts through speaking, writing, and expressive gestures. As Table 1-3 shows, the expressive aphasia disorders go by several diagnostic labels including Broca's, predominantly expressive, motor, non-fluent, and anterior aphasia. Clinically, the verbal encoding disorder is characterized by wordfinding problems, a language disorder, and verbal apraxia (apraxia of speech), a motor speech programming impairment. Agraphia is the expressive encoding disorder affecting writing. The expressive encoding disorder affecting the ability to engage in complicated gestures for communication purposes is referred to as aphasic expressive gestural involvement.

Predominantly Expressive Aphasia

Two clinical features characterize predominantly expressive aphasia seen in Broca's, motor, non-fluent, and anterior aphasia: wordfinding impairments and verbal apraxia. Wordfinding impairments, such as problems recalling words for expression, occur during confrontation naming tasks and during conversational speech. Verbal apraxia, also called apraxia of speech, is impairment of the ability to conceptualize, program, and execute voluntary neuromuscular speech movements. Although each clinical feature may occur independently, both usually occur together in classic aphasias such as those resulting from cerebral vascular accidents. Typically, aphasic patients with predominantly expressive aphasia can be divided into those with a preponderance of wordfinding impairments and those primarily with verbal apraxia symptoms. Patients with a preponderance of wordfinding impairments have more problems recalling words for verbal expression, while those with a predominance of verbal apraxia have more difficulty motorically uttering recalled words.

Wordfinding Impairments

Wordfinding impairments are problems aphasic patients have recalling words to express themselves verbally. Although several diagnostic terms can be used to label this language disorder, such as semantic aphasia, anomia, nominal aphasia, naming deficits, and amnestic aphasia, these terms often have vague and sometimes disparate clinical definitions. Some terms refer to a general category of aphasia or the verbal output seen in some patients with traumatic brain injuries, psychiatric conditions, and dementia. There are seven types of wordfinding behaviors in aphasic patients: mutism, literal phonemic approximations, verbal semantic associations, delay, description, generalization, and tip-of-the-tongue phenomena.

During conversational speech or during confrontation naming exercises, some aphasic patients are mute. When wanting to recall a word during conversation or confronted with the task of labeling or naming something or someone, they cannot conjure any verbal response and are speechless overall or for the particular task. They are wordless to express the particular referent or concept.

Literal phonemic approximation paraphasias occur when the aphasic patient produces a phonemically similar but erroneous word for the desired one; it is a rhyming response. The aphasic patient may say "fell" for "smell," "fun" for "run," or "kun" for "gun." While there are similarities between the struggled attempt to produce a word occurring in verbal apraxia and literal phonemic approximation paraphasias, the latter are phonologically-based and not exclusively a motor programming disorder.

Some aphasic patients may produce verbal semantic association paraphasias during wordfinding behaviors. Verbal semantic association paraphasias occur when the aphasic patient produces a semantically related word for the appropriate one; there is a semantic association. It is an inaccurate circumlocution such as uttering "car" for "truck," "hand" for "foot," or "chair" for "table." Some authorities report "random" naming errors or neologistic paraphasias. Although these do occur, often there is an undiscovered association.

Marshall (1976, p. 446), in a classic study on word retrieval behavior of aphasic adults, identified three additional varieties of wordfinding behaviors: delay, description, and generalization:

> Delay: The patient takes or requests additional time to produce the word. Although some delay is certainly inherent in all retrieval efforts, in this case subjects tended to use a filled pause, unfilled pause, or some stalling tactic to let the listener know they did not want to be interrupted and needed more time to produce the word.

Description: Subjects attempted to produce the desired word by describing what they were talking about. Although associational behaviors were often observed within the context of the subjects' descriptions, the examples … clearly indicate the necessity on the part of the patient to tell something about the intended word.

Generalization: Here subjects produced general words … in place of the desired word. In many instances, this behavior seemed to represent a manipulative effort on part of the aphasic to get the clinician to supply the needed word.

The tip-of-the-tongue phenomenon is what occurs when the patient engages in phonemic and semantic trial-and-error behaviors to find the desired and correct word. In this frustrating behavior, the word appears just out of reach and the patient makes repetitive attempts to say it. The tip-of-the-tongue phenomenon is part of the wordfinding and motor speech production deficits.

Verbal Apraxia

Once the word has been recalled, some patients with predominantly expressive aphasia have difficulty programming it into existence. The patient has the word in his or her internal monologue; he or she has recalled it in inner speech, but programming the neuromuscular actions necessary to produce it is impaired or nonexistent. Verbal apraxia (apraxia of speech) is often seen initially in brain injuries, but because of the reduction of brain edema and other factors, it often subsides or disappears completely.

As discussed previously, verbal apraxia refers to the impaired ability to conceptualize, program, and execute voluntary neuromuscular speech movements. Verbal apraxia primarily affects articulation, but can impair other motor speech processes such as respiration, phonation, and resonance. A key clinical feature of verbal apraxia is automatic speech. Although purposeful and volitional utterances are difficult or impossible to produce, many patients have automatic speech which is sometimes called "subcortical speech." When little thought and attention are given to the utterance, some patients can say over-learned and automatic utterances such as swear words, names of family members, and rote-learned phrases. Patients with predominantly expressive aphasia with a predominance of verbal apraxia have more difficulty voluntarily programming words into existence than recalling them for expression.

In verbal encoding disorders, the output of the aphasic patient is influenced by his or her awareness of errors and ability to self-correct. A patient with awareness of errors knows when she or he has recalled the desired word and produced it correctly. The patient who is self-corrective, through trial and error, can eventually recall and correctly produce the desired word.

The following is an example of predominantly expressive aphasia:

I, swant, uh, want, to say, play, choker; not choker, uh, (pause) choker. No. Poker. I want to say poker today, uh, tonight, with my daught … strife, uh strife, uh, (pause) wife. I bet quarter. Straw choker, uh, uh, foker, uh, forker, forker, puh, orker is game. Damn it, draw poker is my game.

In the above example, the patient displays wordfinding impairments on the words "poker," "today," "wife," and "draw." Verbal apraxia is present on "want," "poker," "wife," and "draw." "Damn it, draw poker is my game" is an example of automatic speech. For the most part, the patient is aware of errors and usually self-corrective.

Aphasic Agraphia

As noted previously, most children are born with the ability to speak using verbal symbols, but humans must be taught to write. Formulating and transforming cognitive information into a written linguistic code is a learned behavior. Written expression shares the essential elements of verbal expression in that it is an arbitrary symbolic representation of reality and is rule-dependent.

Aphasic agraphia is an acquired inability to express oneself in writing not due to arm and hand paralysis. While it is true that many patients with predominantly expressive aphasia may have weak or nonfunctional arms and hands, their core writing problems are not due to paralysis. To illustrate that aphasic agraphia is a disorder of graphic symbolism and not fundamentally a motor problem, patients with severe aphasia cannot meaningfully express themselves in writing even when they hold the pen or pencil in their non-paralyzed hand. Most people can write with their non-dominant hands, albeit with less legibility.

Aphasic patients tend to write like they speak. Patients with fluent jargon write using meaning-less written signs, letters, words, and phrases, which is sometimes referred to as jargon agraphia. Non-fluent patients write haltingly, with many errors of letter form; words are typically misspelled and writing is a perplexing struggle. Since aphasic agraphia is a central graphic language process-ing disorder, spelling impairments usually accompany it.

Although some authorities delineate several different types of acquired agraphia, deep and surface agraphia are the primary writing problems experienced by aphasic patients. Deep agraphia is a problem with written semantic errors and poor phoneme-to-grapheme conversion. Surface agraphia, sometimes called lexical agraphia, results in partial knowledge of written word forms and impaired spelling memory. Benson and Ardila (1996) listed "pure agraphia," writing problems in the absence of other language impairments, as likely occurring as a result of damage to the left premotor cortex.

Aphasic Expressive Gestural Involvement

There are two general types of aphasic expressive gestural impairments that accompany verbal communication: descriptive and reinforcing gestural disorders. A descriptive gesture, as the name implies, involves the speaker using facial, arm, and hand gestures to provide direction or explain an action. Expressive reinforcing gestures are used to emphasize, accentuate, and stress a verbal statement sending information about how the person feels. Expressive gestural communication ranges from simple body movements showing escape and avoidance to complex, language-based gestures involving finger-spelling and sign language. According to Davis (2007), gestures can be evaluated with regard to the transitivity and complexity of body movements. An example of a transitive action on an object is dialing the telephone, and an intransitive action without an object is displaying the "thumbs up" sign. The complexity of gestural expression ranges from single movements, such as pantomiming the drinking of water from a glass, to sequenced gestures, such as showing the steps necessary to get out of bed and go to the bathroom.

Aphasia impairs the ability to communicate ideas through body language and pantomime. This language disorder impairs all modalities of communication including the idea-gesture disconnect in aphasia. Most people with aphasia can express pain, avoidance, escape, and some simple wants and needs through primitive gestures and reactive body movements. Never-the-less, expressing thoughts through elaborate signs and complex pantomime is beyond the capabilities of most patients with this acquired language disorder. Patients with predominantly expressive aphasia have various degrees of impairments expressing themselves using body language and pantomime for expressive purposes. Patients with pure motor speech disorders are more likely to be success-ful using elaborate signs, communication boards, and complex pantomime to express themselves. However, even for patients with pure motor speech disorders, limb apraxia, the inability to engage in purposeful complex body movements, impairs voluntary functional gestural expression.

LANGUAGE DECODING DISORDERS

Language decoding is converting expressed language into an understandable linguistic code, and processing the information cognitively. It is the process by which humans comprehend and

Figure 1-7. Major landmarks of the outer, middle, and inner ear. (Reprinted with permission from Gutman, S. A. [2017.] *Quick Reference Neuroscience,* [3rd ed.]. Thorofare, NJ: SLACK Incorporated.)

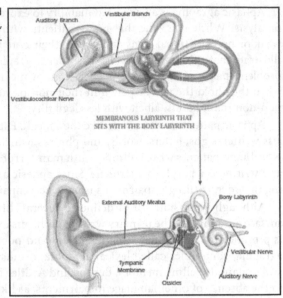

understand the thoughts expressed through speaking, writing, and expressive gestures. Aphasic verbal decoding disorder is the inability to auditorily comprehend spoken language, and alexia is the inability to decode written information. The receptive decoding disorder affecting the ability to understand complicated gestures and pantomime is referred to as "receptive gestural involvement."

Predominately Receptive Aphasia

The aphasic verbal decoding disorder is primarily a disorder of semantics. Patients with this type of aphasia have an inability or reduced ability to comprehend language meaning. In addition, many patients with this predominantly receptive disorder also have fundamental disruptions in the ability to verbally express themselves. This expressive component is called "fluent jargon aphasia."

Auditory Comprehension Disorders

Auditory comprehension of spoken language is dependent on the sense of hearing and auditory perception. The structures of the hearing mechanism transform the acoustic energy generated by the speaker into mechanical, hydraulic, and electrochemical (neural) energy (Figure 1-7). Auditory neural impulses are routed through cranial nerve VIII to the thalamus where the first stage of perception occurs. At the level of the thalamus, elemental meaning is attached to auditory sensation and the perceived salient information is gated to Wernicke's and other areas of the brain. As Figure 1-8 illustrates, the decoding of multiple senses occurs at the posterior multimodal association area. "This posterior multimodal association area integrates sensory information processed by the somatosensory, visual, and auditory association areas, and the olfactory and gustatory cortices" (Gutman, 2008, p. 222). After integration at the posterior multimodal association area, information is sent to the prefrontal cortex (anterior multimodal association area). Higher level decoding and associations of the perceived auditory information involves extracting the denotative and connotative meaning from individual morphemes, words, sentences, phrases, and discourse.

While some authorities persist on defining Wernicke's area of the brain as the "center for auditory comprehension," there is no one "center" for language "comprehension" for these are sophisticated, complicated cognitive functions that engage widespread cortical and subcortical areas of

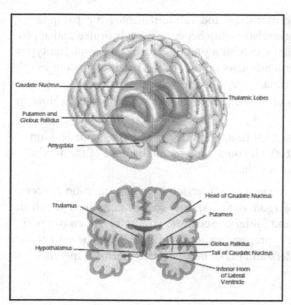

Figure 1-8. Decoding of multiple senses occurs at the posterior multimodal association area. (Reprinted with permission from Gutman, S. A. [2017.] *Quick Reference Neuroscience*, [3rd ed.]. Thorofare, NJ: SLACK Incorporated.)

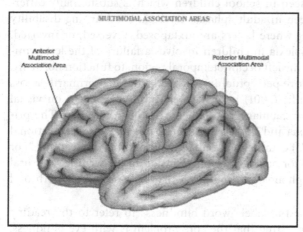

Figure 1-9. Multimodal association areas. (Reprinted with permission from Gutman, S. A. [2017.] *Quick Reference Neuroscience*, [3rd ed.]. Thorofare, NJ: SLACK Incorporated.)

the brain. Perhaps more than any other language function, the process of auditory understanding and comprehension involves the brain operating as a whole and the totality of the mind. "To propose that Wernicke's area of the brain, this small mass of brain cells and the tracts leading to and from it, is the 'center' for verbal 'understanding' … is inexact and inaccurate" (Tanner, 2007, p. 66). Consequently, damage to the Wernicke's area of the brain affects decoding of sensory, perceptual, phonological, grammatical, and the semantic features of language, but only in the context of a cortical conduit to the larger processes of language understanding and comprehension. Figure 1-9 shows the posterior multimodal association area.

Fluent Jargon

Fluent jargon occurs in many patients with the aphasic verbal decoding disorder. Fluent jargon is described as verbalization without semantic substance and is sometimes labeled "word salad" and "logorrhea." In fluent jargon, prosody, rate, rhythm, intonation, stress, and cadence of speech are normal, but the output is semantically impaired or completely lacking in meaningful content. The fluent jargon aphasic patient's output consists of: literal phonemic approximation paraphasias; an alternate word phonemically resembling the desired one; verbal semantic association paraphasias; substitutions with a semantic relationship; and random neologistic paraphasias, where there is no apparent phonemic or semantic relationship between the substituted and appropriate word. Fluent jargon aphasic patients usually exhibit a preponderance of paraphasia types; some patients produce predominantly verbal semantic associations, others produce predominantly literal phonemic approximations, and others primarily random neologistic paraphasias.

The following is an example of fluent jargon in a male patient answering the question: How are you doing?

> The acrylic thus far is preponderance. Tula, est tula, and the acrylic must be made. I am acrylic thus far. Don't you know. (Laughter). Of course, the preponderance of the acrylic is chet jitters and acrylic thus far. So much for that.

In the previous example of jargon aphasia, the patient understood that the question concerns his or her medical condition. The phonemic jargon words, speech sounds combined which do not make sense, are "tula," "est tula," "chet" and "jitters." Semantic jargon, use of conventional words in meaningless context involved "acrylic," "preponderance," and "thus far." The patient also laughed because the listener was unable to understand his or her "perfectly normal" speech.

Aphasic Alexia

Dyslexia is a type of reading problem seen in school children which is substantially different from the reading problems typically seen in adult aphasia. Dyslexia is a learning disability and essentially a visual perceptual disorder where letters are juxtaposed, reversed, or inverted. Shaywitz and Shaywitz (2007) note that dyslexia in children involves a failure of the left-hemisphere posterior brain systems, particularly the left occipitotemporal region, to function normally. Aphasic alexia in adults can include the above perceptual impairments, but it is primarily a loss of written word meanings. Beeson and Hillis (2001) note that reading is dependent on visual analysis of letter strings, graphemic input vocabulary, and letter-to-sound conversion. The primary distinguishing features between dyslexia and aphasic alexia are perceptual and associational impairments. Beeson and Hillis (2001, p. 573) comment on semantic processing and reading: "For example, semantic processing is necessary for auditory comprehension tasks, writing, and oral naming, as well as reading. Similarly, the phonological output lexicon is assessed for both oral naming and oral reading tasks."

Unfortunately, some authorities also use the label "word blindness" to refer to the reading problems seen in patients with aphasia suggesting that the core problem is with eye-blindness. Although strokes, head traumas, and diseases that cause aphasia can also lead to blindness and visual fields deficits, the reading disorder of aphasic alexia is not a result of problems seeing the printed or handwritten word. However, homonymous hemianopsia is a type of visual field deficiency and blindness occurring in neurogenic communication disorders. It is the loss of the same visual half-field of both eyes. Patients are said to have right or left homonymous hemianopsia, which refers to blindness in either the right or left fields of both eyes. Additionally, these patients usually have visual neglect, the lack of awareness of stimuli on the affected side of their bodies.

While patients with aphasic alexia may have cooccurring eye-blindness, homonymous hemianopsia, tunnel vision, and other visual sensory and perceptual deficits, this language decoding disorder is fundamentally a problem semantically decoding written words. Aphasic alexia with agraphia is sometimes referred to as parietal agraphia. As discussed previously, some authorities distinguish between surface and deep (dyslexia) alexia. Surface alexia is a problem "sounding out" written graphemes. Deep alexia involves the patient producing semantic associations when reading aloud. A patient with deep alexia interprets the written word through her or his disordered semantic processor and reads, not the word, but what she or he "thinks" it says, thus producing verbal semantic association paraphasias. The patient may have reduced attention and have difficulty grasping the entire idea of a text. There is a rare reading disorder in neurogenic communication

TABLE 1-4
LANGUAGE ENCODING AND DECODING DISORDERS

LANGUAGE FUNCTION	SYMPTOMS AND MANIFESTATIONS
Language Encoding Impairments	Aphasic Verbal Encoding Disorder (AVED) Wordfinding Impairments Verbal Apraxia Aphasic Agraphia (AA) Aphasic Expressive Gesture Involvement (AEGI)
Language Decoding Impairments	Aphasic Verbal Decoding Disorder (AVDD) Auditory Comprehension Disorders Fluent Jargon Aphasic Alexia (AA) Aphasic Receptive Gestural Involvement (ARGI)

disorders called alexia without agraphia. In this disorder, the patient has trouble reading, but writing is done relatively well. Remarkably, some patients with alexia without agraphia cannot read what they have just written.

Aphasic Receptive Gestural Involvement

The aphasic gestural communication problem discussed in the section on language encoding disorders is not limited to the patient's inability to express himself or herself through gesture and pantomime; it is also a gestural understanding and comprehension disorder. Comprehending gestures ranges from grasping the intent of simple one-movement hand actions, such as beckoning someone using the index finger, to making sense of complex pantomimes and appreciating the nuances of interpretative dance. It also includes appreciating the nonverbal effects of facial expression. This impairment is referred to as aphasic receptive gestural involvement.

Impairment of understanding and comprehending gestural communication in aphasic patients is associated with other language-based disorders. Aphasic naming deficits, auditory comprehension disorders, and general language impairments correlate with impaired pantomime recognition. There is also a strong relationship between reading and pantomime comprehension disorders.

Understanding gestures, particularly regarding nonverbal communication and emotion, and the interpretation of visual-spatial-temporal physical actions, involve the right hemisphere of the brain. However, the idea that the right hemisphere of the brain has entirely different functions regarding interpreting emotions and gestures is misleading. The two hemispheres of the brain are involved in almost every processing task.

Cortical representation of prepositions provides a good example of bi-hemispheric and visual-spatial-temporal brain functions. Conventional brain-based learning models and linguistic localization theories postulate language as a left-hemisphere phenomenon in most people. However, with just a moment's thought, it must be recognized that prepositional concepts such as "in," "beside," "below," "above," and so forth are as much visual-spatial-temporal concepts as linguistic ones. The same is true for interpreting gestures as linguistic symbols. Table 1-4 classifies and summarizes the encoding and decoding disorders in aphasia.

PSYCHOLOGY OF APHASIA AND EFFICACY OF THERAPY

Over the past 50 years, there have been more than two hundred studies conducted of the efficacy of therapy for patients with aphasia and related disorders. While most research shows therapies for aphasia are effective and worthwhile for speech and language recovery, they also suggest they are valuable psychologically. For both patients and family members, the support, direction, and guidance provided by clinicians are important, if not necessary, to optimal recovery. This places a premium on clinicians being aware of the multiple psychological factors associated with aphasia. Unfortunately, the psychology of aphasia is often a neglected academic and clinical subject in most college and university training programs for communication sciences and disorders. For example, while clinicians must learn much about the neurology of communication disorders, of which they can do nothing to change for the patient, the psychology of aphasia is addressed minimally or neglected altogether. As reported previously, most aphasia textbooks relegate the psychological aspects of these disorders to the end of the book almost as an incidental afterthought. A half century ago, Schuell, Jenkins, and Jimenez-Pabon (1964, p. 315) in their classic text, *Aphasia in Adults,* addressed the importance of the psychology of aphasia:

> To say a clinician must be aware of psychological problems in aphasia is to say he must be aware that he is dealing with people. Sometimes we are so intimidated by labels, such as emotional lability, catastrophic reactions, anxiety, depression, euphoria, etc., that we forget this first principle. We talk trade jargon with glibness that betrays our dearth of insights. We talk as though aphasic patients were different from everyone else, and we had to have a different set of rules for dealing with them.

According to Tetnowski (2009, p. ix): "Psychological issues can have an impact on otherwise clear, understandable diagnoses. If we are to treat the whole person, we must understand the importance of psychological factors surrounding neurogenic communication disorders."

Sigmund Freud addressed aphasia and the unconscious mind. However, as reported previously, John Hughlings Jackson, considered by many to be the father of British neurology, was the first to systematically study aphasia and related disorders from a psychological perspective. Jackson proposed a unitary, psychological approach to the study of aphasia. Jackson addressed the idea of inner speech and applied it to aphasia. Jackson did not artificially separate the aphasia patient's psyche from his or her cognition, speech, and language processes, and his or her intent during communication. Since Jackson's groundbreaking work on the psychology of aphasia, three issues have evolved that continue to challenge scientists and clinicians: psycho-organic factors, loss of verbal defense mechanisms, and the grief response.

MAJOR PSYCHOLOGICAL ISSUES IN APHASIA

While most psychological issues discussed next primarily occur in aphasia, they can also occur in motor speech disorders such as apraxia of speech and dysarthrias. Each of these issues affect the quality-of-life of people with aphasia and other neurogenic communication disorders.

The first issue in the psychology of aphasia concerns brain and nervous system damage. It has long been known that certain psychological, emotional, and behavioral reactions occur because of brain and nervous system damage. These psychological, emotional, and behavioral reactions range from depression to euphoria. Scientists and clinicians are currently investigating the relationships of these psychological, emotional, and behavioral reactions to the nature and extent of the neurological damage.

The second issue currently being addressed in aphasia concerns psychological defenses and coping styles. All people use defense mechanisms and coping styles to deal with anxiety and stress. Some defense mechanisms and coping styles are mature, adaptive, and lead to good mental health

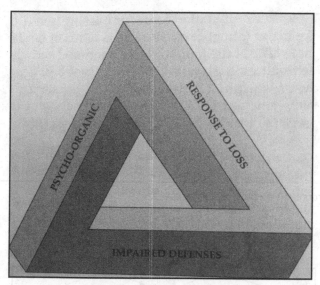

Figure 1-10. Three factors to the psychology of aphasia.

while others are immature, radical, and desperate attempts to deal with unpleasantness. Patients with aphasia employ them with differing degrees of success as a consequence of the impairments of language. Of particular interest is how the loss of language seen in people with aphasia affects these defense mechanisms and coping styles. Some defense mechanisms and coping styles are nonverbal, such as denial, while others are verbal, such as rationalization. Aphasic patients can be deprived of many verbal defense mechanisms due to their loss of language.

The third psychological issue concerns how patients cope with unwanted change. People with aphasia often experience permanent separation from abilities, loved ones, and valued objects. These patients, like all persons, can be expected to grieve over those losses and to pass through predictable stages of accepting unwanted changes. While there is individual variability in these grieving stages, and special issues associated with impaired or lost abilities to communicate, most patients with aphasia feel a deep sense of loss. They grieve over the loss of physical abilities, valued objects, and breakdown in communication with loved ones.

While there is overlap in the above three aspects of the psychology of aphasia, each of them, more or less, play a role in the patient's psychology and adjustment to the disability. Some patients are more psychologically affected by the brain and nervous system damage. Other patients experience more grief reactions, and still others, such as global aphasics, have reduced abilities to cope due to the loss of verbal psychological defenses and coping styles. Many neurogenic communication disorders are major life-altering events, and understanding the patient's psychology is fundamental to helping him or her return to a meaningful and fulfilling quality-of-life. As noted previously, serious medical conditions often cause aphasia, bringing on many adjustment challenges, and the language disorder can sever communication between the patient and those who can and want to help with recovery and adjustment. Figure 1-10 shows the three issues in the psychology of aphasia. The variable influence of each factor among individual patients is illustrated by Figure 1-11.

Aphasia and Quality-of-Life

Although quality-of-life is an important topic when addressing the human experience, it is rarely defined. When discussing quality-of-life, most people simply assume there is a general consensus about what it is for all people, at all ages, and under all circumstances. There is a general belief that what is a good or poor quality-of-life for one person will be the same for another. In fact,

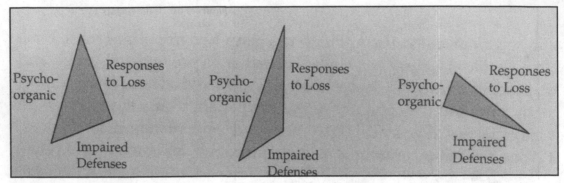

Figure 1-11. Variable influences of the three factors in the psychology of aphasia.

Figure 1-12. Lawton's conceptual model of quality of life.

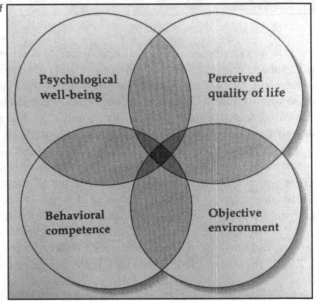

the factors that contribute or detract from quality-of-life are highly variable. One person's idea of a good quality-of-life may be viewed as an impoverished and unsatisfying existence by another.

Lawton (1991) defines quality-of-life as having four critical domains which interact with each other: psychological well-being, perceived quality-of-life, behavioral competence, and objective environment (Figure 1-12). Communication competence is a necessary component in the four critical domains.

Psychological Well-Being

A person must be free of mental illness to experience a good quality-of-life. No one would argue that having a good quality-of-life is impossible for a person who is in the grips of a deep depression or suffering from frequent panic attacks. However, a sense of psychological well-being is more than being free from mental illness. It is also having a reason to live, optimism about life in general, spiritual meaningfulness, and social contacts with whom to share life's journey. Underlying this sense of well-being are the brain chemicals serotonin and dopamine. When these chemicals are in proper balance they are biological agents that contribute to a positive emotional state.

The opposite of a sense of psychological well-being is depression. To some neuroscientists and clinicians, non-grieving depression is an imbalance of chemicals in the brain. To some mental health authorities, people get depressed-anxious because they do not produce "feel good" chemicals in adequate amounts or they are eliminated too quickly from the body. The result is having an inadequate level of these chemicals causes various degrees of depression. The medical treatment for depression is the administration of antidepressants. The current generation of antidepressants results in higher levels of these mood enhancing chemicals in the patient's brain and, for the most part, they are remarkably free of serious side-effects in adults. In aphasia, the depression seen in many patients is caused by a chemical imbalance resulting from damage to specific areas of the brain and nervous system.

A social and psychotherapeutic explanation for depression is that it is primarily stress-induced. It is common for a person to experience high levels of stress preceding or during the onset of the depression. According to the American Psychiatric Association (2013, p. 829), a stressor is "Any emotional, physical, economic, or other factor that disrupts the normal physiological, cognitive emotional, or behavior balance of an individual." The stress can be positive or negative. For example, loss of a job is a negative stressor, while being promoted to a new one can be a positive stressor. The relationship between stress and depression is highly variable and what one person finds stressful another may not. When under chronic stress, some people feel depressed, hopeless, and helpless. Through counseling, exercise, and psychotherapy, depressed people can learn to cope with stress and depression.

While it may seem that the above chemical and stress explanations for a sense of psychological well-being are unrelated, they may be integrally tied to each other. An individual's non-adaptive way of dealing with stress may cause a reduction in serotonin and other mood enhancing brain chemicals. In effect stress, and a person's inability properly to deal with it, may cause brain chemistry to go awry. Because of this brain-mind relationship, most treatments of depression involve counseling, psychotherapy and the administration of antidepressants, if necessary.

For most people, communication competence is necessary for a sense of psychological well-being. Most people need to be able to communicate with others about important aspects of their lives and the emotions associated with life changes. In addition, counseling and psychotherapy are "talking cures" for depression and other psychopathologies. For individuals with aphasia, their significant communication disorder can create barriers to overcoming depression and a reduced sense of psychological well-being.

Perceived Quality-of-Life

As reported above, perceived quality-of-life is a subjective estimate and differs from one person to another. If one perceives he or she is experiencing a good quality-of-life, this belief actually contributes to it. Conversely, if a person feels that her or his life is impoverished, this perception contributes to a poor quality-of-life. Other than health, there are few objective events or situations that are universally perceived to contribute to quality-of-life. Even wealth is not necessarily associated with a high quality of living. Perception of one's quality-of-life is fundamentally tied to a person's self-esteem.

Self-esteem is a positive belief and feeling about one's self. As noted previously, Joseph Wepman, an early aphasiologist, observed that in all instances of brain damage, there is some reduction in the patient's self-esteem. For people with aphasia, their previous beliefs and attitudes about people with disabilities will affect their self-esteem and quality-of-life. Brumfitt (1996) observed that an aphasic patient's identity must change based on the new disability.

Perceived quality-of-life is also affected by the way patients adapt to chronic illness. According to LaPointe (1997), successful adaptation to chronic illness involves going from uncertainty to regaining wellness through taking charge, setting goals, seeking closure, and attaining mastery over the illness. The patient's communication competence is important to successful adaptation to disabilities and regaining a positive perceived quality-of-life. Positive perceptions of the patient's aphasia can be facilitated by doctors, nurses, therapists, and others involved with the patient's rehabilitation.

Behavioral Competence

Behavioral competence is the patient's ability to exercise control over his or her environment. People who can exert control over their lives are less likely to suffer from depression and the hopelessness and helplessness that often accompany it. For patients with neurogenic communication disorders, the physical disabilities often accompanying these disorders can limit behavioral competence. Hemiparalysis which often cooccurs with aphasia is a significant deterrent to behavioral competence.

Hemiparalysis affects behavioral competence particularly in regard to activities of daily living. Hemiparalysis can disrupt or eliminate the patient's ability to walk, dress, eat, groom, and independently go to the bathroom. These limitations dramatically affect the patient's quality-of-life. Regaining wellness and attaining mastery over disability is due to the success of occupational, vocational, and physical therapies in addressing the hemiparalysis.

Perhaps the most significant behavioral competence limitations are neurogenic communication disorders that render patients functionally unable to communicate. Communication is the primary way people exercise control over their environments. Whether it is a business executive directing the course of his or her corporation through communication with subordinates, or a husband and wife negotiating the responsibilities of child care, communication is indispensable to exercising control of one's affairs. Significant neurogenic communication disorders can deprive patients with even a modicum of control over their environments. To show the importance of functional communication on quality-of-life, in a study addressing laryngeal cancer, MacNeil, Weischselbaum, and Pauker (1981) found that most of the subjects were willing to trade off life expectancy to retain the ability to speak. For patients with aphasia, achieving any degree of functional speech and language or utilizing alternative communication systems are essential to regaining a good quality-of-life.

Objective Environment

Some people with aphasia are institutionalized. The quality of long-term rehabilitation centers, nursing homes, and other extended care facilities vary greatly and can significantly affect a patient's quality-of-life. Some facilities provide optimal long-term services to disabled persons that contribute to high quality living. At these facilities, the food is healthy and patients receive a balanced diet, there are recreational activities, reading rooms, media centers, solariums, clubs, sports, exercise programs, and the medical, nursing, and rehabilitation programs in these facilities are of the highest quality. Unfortunately, there are other facilities that do not provide the necessary objective environment for quality living.

The objective environment for patients who return home also varies greatly. Some objective home environments are loving, healthy, stimulating, and provide more than the essentials to achieving a high quality-of-life for the patient. Many patients are positively reintegrated into the family roles and responsibilities reflecting their abilities to communicate. As with long-term care institutions, there are also patients who return to a home where the objective environment is far less than optimal and detracts from quality living. A barometer of the objective environment is the quality of communication occurring with the patient and health care professionals.

Stress and Aphasia

Stress is a core aspect of all major neurogenic communication disorders. The stressors associated with neurogenic communication disorders are varied and unique to each patient and can significantly affect quality-of-life. Listed below are common stressors associated with aphasia and related disorders:

- Being psychologically separated from loved ones due to a communication disorder
- Difficulty understanding the speech of others
- Experiencing a medical emergency
- Impairments with walking, eating, dressing, and going to the bathroom
- Knowledge that you have experienced brain damage
- Medical expenses
- Medications
- New relationships with doctors, nurses, and therapists
- Physical separation from loved ones for long periods
- Problems doing simple arithmetic
- Reading deficits
- Slurred speech
- Suffering a serious neurological event
- Tip-of-the-tongue behaviors
- Undergoing MRI, CT, video swallowing studies, and other diagnostic tests
- Wordfinding deficits

A particular person's reaction to stress is determined by premorbid personality traits such as perfectionism, compulsivity, and overly critical concerns about other people's evaluations of him or her. When it comes to adapting to aphasia, stress plays two important roles. First, stress places a demand on coping skills. The patient's previously learned and automatic psychological adjustment strategies are taxed as he or she attempts to cope with a myriad of stressful events. The patient's ongoing attempts to adjust to major illness, physical and psychological separation from loved ones, financial woes, frustrating attempts at communication, and mental and physical limitations can overwhelm previously successful adjustment strategies. As reported previously, stress is a risk factor in major depression. Stuart (1998) noted that the average depressed person reports three times as many important life events during the six months prior to the onset of clinical depression than did normal subjects. Over time, the cumulative effects of the unwanted changes can exceed the patient's ability to adjust to them.

Second, the inability to cope can also be a stressor. The patient's slow, frustrating, and often unsuccessful ability to adjust can create a perception that the brain injury has eliminated his or her previously successful coping abilities. Particularly in the case of depression, this can lead to overwhelming feelings of helplessness and hopelessness. For some patients, not only have they been overwhelmed by stress, but they have the sense that the brain injury itself has eliminated the ability to ever regain psychological stability. Hilari, Cruice, Sorin-Peters, and Worrall (2015) observe that to improve quality-of-life in aphasic patients, interventions should also promote emotional well-being, strengthening social networks, and social participation in addition to treatment of the communication disorder.

Case Studies, Illustrations, and Examples: Stress and the Evaluation

You are wheeled into a sterile, but comfortable office. As a woman locks your wheelchair in place and engages in chitchat, you occasionally nod, provide slanted smiles, and utter "uh, huh" at the end of her statements. Only fragments of her speech are understood by you. The next hour is spent pointing to pictures, opening your mouth widely, writing, sticking out your tongue, and putting small red circles below large green squares. Scores of your responses, actions, and behaviors are noted carefully by the clinician. At the end of this emotionally draining hour, you are painfully aware of every defect, deficit, deficiency, deviation, and disorder in your once normal ability to communicate. Despair huddles on the horizon as you begin to let the reality of your predicament set in.

In the report, the words "spastic dysarthria" labels the inability to make your vocal cords vibrate easily and freely; your voice sounds as though hands are tightly choking your neck. So, too, do those medical words describe your tongue's slow, sluggish, and restricted movements. The sounds of speech, in the past so easily and automatically produced, are now made with distortions, slurs, and imprecision. Your speech muscles are weak, sluggish participants in the act of talking. Paralyzed muscles make your face rigid, and even when you can force a phony smile, they betray your intent.

"Apraxia of speech" in the diagnostic report could better be called impotence ... verbal impotence. As occasional words surface to your mind's ear, attempts to utter them are met with resistance. Try as you will, you can't seem to remember how to shape the air coming from your lungs into speech. The in and out of breathing resists formation into words. When you attempt a word, when you carefully think about its creation, you fail to complete or even start the act. It is as though the word has no trigger to fire it into existence. You feel not confused, but perplexed. When flawed words emerge from your mouth, they cause your stomach to tighten. You feel out-of-control. It is frightening to have speech muscles with minds of their own. What is even more perplexing is the occasional utterance that flows from your mouth with ease. Like swear words that surface when your thumb is crushed by a hammer, these automatic utterances are programmed into existence when no thought is given to them. The clinician notes the presence of "automatic" speech on your report. What has not been noted is your overwhelming sense of impotence, the loss of psychological integrity, and completeness of what was once you.

"Aphasia." A rose by any other name would still have thorns capable of piercing your sense of self. Where have the words gone? Where are the lost verbal trains of thought stationed? It is as though a vacuum has sucked away so many of the little and large words that once resided in your mind. What has happened to the "readin," "writin," and "rithmetic" you learned so many years ago in school?

As you stare intently at the nameless object carefully placed on the table by the clinician, you try and try to remember its name. Oh sure, you know it is for grooming. With your left hand, you could easily grasp it, and pull it through your hair. Its color, shape, and function are familiar, but its name escapes you. "Tooth?" No, that didn't sound right. "Brush?" No, well, maybe. "Comb." It is a Comb! One down, thousands to go. As the hour crawls on, you confront one failure after another while only occasionally satisfying the demanding clinician.

"Point to the fork"

"Show me the one used for eating"

"Read this word"

"Write the name of this, that, and the other thing"

"Fill in the blank"

"Complete this sentence"

"Remember this word"

"Construct this sentence"

"Choose the correct one"

"Tell me"

"Speak to me"

"Talk, talk, talk"

Finally, the evaluation and psychological trauma are over. Whew! Now, you will be defined, described, and diagnosed. The how's, what's, when's, and where's of rehabilitation will be neatly fit into the Medicare and HMO's service standards. Fortunately for you, and unfortunately for the diagnostic report, your communication disorders, and your feelings about them, will change and evolve. Some of what was discovered today will be irrelevant next week and much of the report will be obsolete next month. But let the games begin. You now have a new identity, a new role. You are now just one of many patients to the therapist. Feelings of inferiority build.

CHAPTER SUMMARY

Aphasia can dramatically and negatively affect all four domains of a person's quality-of-life: psychological well-being, perceived quality-of-life, behavioral competence, and objective environment. Depression, anxiety, and a host of other negative psychological states, can profoundly reduce a patient's psychological well-being. In addition, the person's behavioral competence and perceived quality-of-life can be reduced and the communication disorder can interfere with the quality of his or her objective environment. While therapies for aphasia and related disorders have been proven to be beneficial in recovering speech and language abilities, addressing the psychology of these disorders by all health care professionals can improve the quality-of-life of most patients.

REFERENCES

American Psychiatric Association. (2013). *Diagnostic and statistical manual of mental disorders* (5th ed.). Arlington, VA: American Psychiatric Association.

Baker, M., and Tanner, D. (1990). *Recovery from brain insult: Investigation of patient and family adaptation*. Paper presented at the annual convention of the Canadian Association of Speech-Language Pathologists and Audiologists, Vancouver, BC.

Beeson, P. M., and Hillis, A. E. (2001). Comprehension and production of written words. In R. Chapey (Ed.), *Language intervention in aphasia and related neurogenic communication disorders* (4th ed.). Philadelphia, PA: Lippincott Williams and Wilkins.

Benson, F. D., and Ardila, A. (1996). *Aphasia: A clinical perspective*. New York, NY: Oxford University Press.

Brain, R. (1965). *Speech disorders: Aphasia, apraxia and agnosia* (2nd ed.). Washington, DC: Butterworth.

Brumfitt, S. (1996). Losing your sense of self: What aphasia can do. In C. Code (Ed.), *Forums in clinical aphasiology* (pp. 349-355). London, UK: Whurr.

Campbell, J. (1982). *Grammatical man: Information, entropy, language, and life*. New York, NY: Simon and Schuster.

Critchley, M. (1970). *Aphasiology and other aspects of language*. London, UK: Edward Arnold.

Darley, F. (1982). *Aphasia*. Philadelphia: Saunders.

Davis, G.A. (2007). *Aphasiology: Disorders and clinical practice* (2nd ed.). Boston, MA: Pearson, Allyn and Bacon.

Eisenson, J. (1984). *Adult aphasia*, (2nd ed.). Englewood Cliffs, NJ: Prentice-Hall.

Fridriksson, J., Fillmore, P., Dazhou, G., and Rorden, C. (2015). Chronic Broca's aphasia is caused by damage to Broca's and Wernicke's areas. *Cerebral Cortex, 25*(12), 4689-4696.

Gutman, S. (2008). *Quick reference neuroscience for rehabilitation professionals*. Thorofare, NJ: Slack.

Head, H. (1926). *Aphasia and kindred disorders of speech*. Cambridge, UK: Cambridge University Press.

Hilari, K., Cruice, M., Sorin-Peters, R., and Worrall, L. (2015). Quality of life in aphasia: State of the art. *Folia Phoniatrica et Logopaedica.* 67 (3): 114-118.

Itabashi, R., Yoshiyuki, N., Kataoka, Y., Yazawi, Y., Furui, E., Minoru, M., and Mori, E. (2015). Damage to the left precentral gyrus is associated with apraxia of speech in acute stroke. *Stroke.* 47 (1): 31-36.

Jackson, J. (1878). On affections of speech from diseases of the brain. *Brain.* 1: 301-330.

Laakso, M. (2003). Collaborative construction of repair in aphasic conversation: An interactive view on the extended speaking turns of persons with Wernicke's Aphasia. In C. Goodwin (Ed). *Conversation and brain damage* (pp. 163-188). Oxford, UK: Oxford University Press.

LaPointe, L. (1997). Adaptation, accommodation, aristos. In L. LaPointe (Ed.), *Aphasia and related neurogenic language disorders* (2nd ed.). New York, NY: Thieme.

Lawton, M. (1991). A multidimensional view of quality of life in frail elders. In J. Birren (Ed.), *The concept and measurement of quality of life in frail elders.* San Diego, CA: Academic Press.

MacNeil, B., Weischselbaum, R., and Pauker, S. (1981). Speech and survival: Tradeoffs between quality and quality of life in laryngeal cancer. *New England Journal of Medicine,* 305 (17): 983-987.

Marshall, R. (1976). Word retrieval behavior of aphasic adults. *Journal of Speech and Hearing Disorders,* 41: 444-451.

Pachaiska, M., Jastrzebowska, G., Gryglicka, K., Mirska, N., and Macqueen, B. (2015) Distrubances of communication in persons with traumatic brain injury. *Acta Neuropsychologica,* 13(2): 105-125.

Sarno, J. (1981). Emotional aspects of aphasia. In M. Sarno (Ed.), *Acquired aphasia.* New York, NY: Academic Press.

Sarno, M. (1991). Treatment of aphasia workshop research and research needs. *Aphasia treatment: Current approaches and research opportunities,* 2, xi-xvi.

Schuell, H., Jenkins, J., and Jimenez-Pabon, E. (1964). *Aphasia in adults.* New York, NY: Harper and Row.

Scott, K., and Tanner, D. (1990). *Recovery from brain insult: Investigation of patient adaptation and recovery.* Paper presented at the annual convention of the Canadian Association of Speech-Language Pathologists and Audiologists, Vancouver, BC.

Shaywitz, S., and Shaywitz, B. (2007). The neurobiology of reading and dyslexia. *ASHA Leader,* 12 (12), 20-21.

Sternberg, R., and Ben-Zeev, T. (2001). *Complex cognition: The psychology of human thought.* New York, NY: Oxford University Press.

Stuart, G. (1998). Self-concept responses and dissociative disorders. In G. Stuart and M. Laraia (Eds.), *Principles and practice of psychiatric nursing* (6th ed.). St. Louis, MO: Mosby.

Tanner, D. (2006). *An advanced course in communication sciences and disorders.* San Diego, CA: Plural.

Tanner, D. (2007). Redefining Wernicke's area: Receptive language and discourse semantics. *Journal of Allied Health,* 36 (2):63-66.

Tetnowski, J. (2009). Foreword. In D. Tanner, *The psychology of neurogenic communication disorders: A primer for health care professionals.* New York, NY: iUniverse.

Vygotsky, L. (1962). *Thought and language.* New York, NY: MIT Press and John Wiley & Sons.

Wepman, J. (1962). The language disorders. In J. F. Garrett and E. S. Levine (Eds.), *Psychological practices with the physically disabled.* New York, NY: Colombia University Press.

Weisenburg, T., and McBride, K. (1935). *Aphasia.* New York, NY: Commonwealth Fund.

Psychology of Aphasia and Brain Damage

"Language is not simply a reporting device for experience but a defining framework for it."

Benjamin Lee Whorf

CHAPTER PREVIEW

This chapter examines the psycho-organic determinants of aphasia and related disorders. Brain damage is considered a predisposing factor in the many psychological reactions and disorders seen in people with aphasia; although brain damage can also precipitate and perpetuate these reactions and disorders. In this chapter, the psychological reactions and disorders based on the type and location of brain damage seen in patients with aphasia and related disorders are explored. This chapter covers emotional lability, catastrophic reactions, perseveration, organic depression-anxiety disorder, anosognosia, homonymous hemianopsia, visual neglect, and euphoria. Also addressed are the behavioral and adjustment problems seen in some patients with traumatic brain injuries.

BRAIN DAMAGE AS A PREDISPOSING FACTOR IN THE PSYCHOLOGY OF APHASIA

The role brain damage plays in the psychology of aphasia has been studied for decades. Today a great deal of research is being conducted on the site of brain injury associated with or causing psychological reactions and disorders. The goal is to identify areas of the brain causing psychosis, aggression, denial, depression, euphoria, and many other psychological reactions and disorders. Strict localizationists (associationists) believe that all significant psychological reactions and disorders can be traced to specific parts of the brain and that depression, anxiety, psychosis, and so forth, are directly caused by brain injury. Other scientists and clinicians, gestaltists (cognitivists), acknowledge that injury to parts of the brain are associated with many psychological reactions and disorders, but they are not the absolute cause of them. A good example of the localization versus holistic view of the psycho-organic determinants of the psychology of aphasia is clinical depression.

To strict localizationists, clinical depression seen in patients with aphasia is a direct result of damage to specific parts of the brain. As discussed in Chapter 1, brain damage causes a deficiency of certain neurochemicals associated with a sense of well-being, and results in depression often accompanied by anxiety. The treatment for this psycho-organic depression is the administration of antidepressants which correct the neurochemical imbalance. Gestaltists, on the other hand, acknowledge the role brain damage plays in the onset of clinical depression in patients with aphasia, but also consider the role stress, loss, grief, and coping styles and defense mechanisms play in clinical depression. Gestaltists believe antidepressants should be combined with counseling, psychotherapy, lifestyle changes, exercise, and other social treatments for depression. Some authorities label the localization school of thought, the medical model, while the gestaltist philosophy is sometimes referred to as cognitivists and the social model. Currently, much research is being conducted into these issues often with controversial and inconclusive results.

When addressing the psycho-organic determinants in the psychology of aphasia, the predisposing, precipitating, and perpetuating factors associated with brain injury must be addressed to explain the adjustment challenges and psychological reactions and disorders experienced by some patients. Although brain damage may precipitate and perpetuate psychological disorders and maladjustment to aphasia, it is best viewed as a predisposing factor. A precipitating factor is an important or necessary condition to cause a psychological disorder or to set a maladaptive response into motion. A perpetuating factor causes the psychological reaction or disorder to be persistent or permanent. The predisposing factor(brain damage) incline a patient to a particular psychological condition, attitude, or behavior.

Due to brain damage, patients with aphasia can be predisposed to certain psychological reactions and disorders. A good example of the predisposing influence of temporal lobe damage is aggressive, violent, and impulsive behavior. Temporal lobe epilepsy is associated with purposeless violence, and has even been used as a defense in legal cases (Tanner, 2007). Some legal authorities have proposed that violent offenders have inherited brain irregularities leading to a propensity for criminal behavior. As with most localization research, studies addressing aggressive, violent, and impulsive behavior often result in disparate and sometimes contradictory results. Frontal lobe damage has also been linked to aggressive, violent, impulsive, and other antisocial behaviors. However, it is well-documented that brain injury can predispose a person for certain dissocial behaviors. Importantly, it should be noted that while some individuals with temporal and frontal lobe damage become violent offenders, most do not. Consequently, psycho-organic determinants are best viewed as predisposing factors requiring precipitating, perpetuating, and other yet to be discovered phenomena to account for maladjustment and psychological disorders in aphasia.

GENERALITIES ABOUT BRAIN INJURY AND PSYCHOLOGICAL REACTIONS AND DISORDERS

Certain generalities can be made about the nature, type, and location of brain injury and their predisposing effects for certain psychological reactions and disorders in patients with neurogenic communication disorders (American Psychiatric Association, 2013; Black, 1975; Carota, Rossetti, Karapanayiotides, and Bogousslavsky, 2001; Gainotti, 1972, 1989; Gasparini, Satz, Heilman, and Coolidge, 1978; Gordon, Hibbard, Egelko, and Diller, 1985; Gordon, Hibbard, and Morganstein, 1996; Lipsey, Spencer, Rabins, and Robinson, 1986; Robinson, Boston, Starkstein, and Price, 1988;

TABLE 2-1
TYPE AND LOCATION OF BRAIN INJURY AND PSYCHOLOGICAL GENERALITIES

PSYCHOLOGICAL DEFENSE AND COPING STYLE	DESCRIPTION
Traumatic Brain Injury	Neuropsychological deficits not typically seen in stroke including: • Posttraumatic Psychosis • Amnesia and Disorientation • Behavior Disorders Differences in open and closed head injury symptoms initially with diverging manifestation overtime
Stroke	Long-Lasting Depression
Left-Hemisphere Damage	Anxiety Depression
Right-Hemisphere Damage	Indifference Apathy Cheerfulness Euphoria
Posterior Left-Hemisphere	Indifference Anosognosia Euphoria
Anterior Left-Hemisphere	Anxiety Depression
Wernicke's Area	Anosognosia Indifference Euphoria
Broca's Area	Short-Lived Emotional Outbursts Anxiety Depression

Robinson, 1986; Robinson, et al., 1985; Robinson and Benson, 1981; Sackeim, et al., 1982; Sackeim and Weber, 1982; Smeltzer, Nasrallah, and Miller, 1994; Tanner, 2007, 2009, 2010; Tanner and Gerstenberger, 1996; Tardiff, 1997; Weinstein, Lyerly, Cole, and Ozer, 1966; Weinstein and Puig-Antich, 1974; Williams, Evans, and Fleminger, 2003; Ylvisaker, Szekeres, and Feeney, 2001). It is important to note that many adjustment challenges and psychological disorders predisposed by brain injury are not substantially different from the kinds of reactions and disorders seen in psychologically disturbed people without brain damage (functional disorders).

As Table 2-1 illustrates, traumatic brain injury is associated with cognitive, memory, learning, and orientation deficits not typically seen in strokes. Initially, open and closed head injuries tend to

Figure 2-1. Approximate sites in the brain associated with psychological reactions in some patients with neurogenic communication disorders.

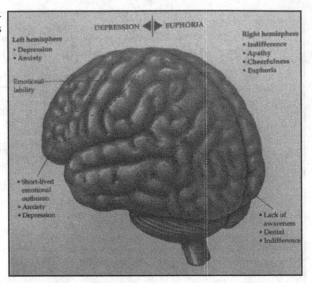

present with similar psychological symptoms, but as time passes, they diverge in their symptomatology. Approximately 50% of people who have communication disorders resulting from stroke will experience long-lasting depression. Regardless of etiology, patients with left-hemisphere brain damage are predisposed to anxiety and depression, while those suffering right-hemisphere injuries are more likely to be indifferent, apathetic, cheerful, and even euphoric. When the brain injury is in the posterior part of the left hemisphere, patients are predisposed to indifference, anosognosia (lack of awareness or denial of disability), and euphoria. When the brain injury is to the anterior part of the left-hemisphere, as many as 70% of patients are likely to experience depression often accompanied by anxiety. Damage to Wernicke's area predisposes patients to anosognosia. Damage to Broca's area is associated with short-lived emotional outbursts, anxiety, and depression. Smaller brain lesions generally result in more awareness of disability than larger ones, likely contributing to the patient's frustration, anxiety, and depression. Figure 2-1 depicts the approximate location of certain psychological reactions and disorders in some patients with neurogenic communication disorders.

PERSEVERATION AND ECHOLALIA

Perseveration is the tendency for a person inappropriately to continue an act for a longer duration than is warranted by the significance of the stimulus that prompted it. According to the American Psychiatric Association (2013), perseveration is an aspect of the personality trait domain Negative Affectivity. Echolalia, a manifestation of perseveration, is where a patient automatically repeats the sound, word, or phrase spoken by someone else. Mitigated echolalia, a normal process, is when a person repeats the last thing spoken by someone else when bidding for time to process the information. Psychologically, echolalic responses occur in many patients to fill silences and to give the appearance of normalcy. Perseveration and echolalia are seen in patients with aphasia arising from stroke, traumatic brain injury, and degenerative neurological diseases. In perseveration, the patient appears to be stuck in a rigid mental set and cannot shift to an appropriate one. Kaplan, Gallagher, and Glosser (1998) considered perseveration an intrusive interference of previous responses and problematic for many aphasic patients.

Perseveration has been likened to a song normal people continue to process after the stimulus that prompted it has ceased. This occurrence in normal people, however, is not as intense as what occurs in patients with aphasia, and can be ceased relatively easily by distraction and shifts in attention.

Sandson and Albert (1984, p. 715) proposed three types of perseveration and identify sites of lesions associated with them: stuck-in-set, recurrent, and continuous.

Stuck-in-set perseveration, the inappropriate maintenance of a current category or framework, involves an underlying process deficit in executive functioning and is related neuroanatomically to frontal lobe damage. Recurrent perseveration, the unintentional repetition of a previous response to a subsequent stimulus, involves an abnormal post-facilitation of memory traces and is related neuroanatomically to posterior left hemisphere damage. Continuous perseveration is the inappropriate prolongation or repetition of a behavior without interruption. It involves a deficit in motor output and is most common in patients with damage to the basal ganglia.

Perseveration behaviors typically occur in two modalities in aphasic patients: verbal and graphic. An example of verbal perseveration is the patient repeating the same response to an initial question when others are asked. For example, in sentence completion therapy, the patient may respond to the request to complete the statement, "Red, white, and _____," with the correct verbal response: "blue." The perseveration response occurs when the patient also responds with "blue" to the following: "Knife, fork, and _____," and "The United States of _____." According to Morganstein and Smith (2001, p. 388), perseveration can be highly problematic in therapy:

Typically, this tendency is discovered once treatment is underway and the clinician observes that the patient's responses, rather than demonstrating the advances in vocabulary retrieval and sentence use, contain recycled errors in word choices which are not evolving into something better.

Graphic perseveration occurs when the patient's writing begins correctly, but then degenerates to repeated letters often trailing off to a straight line.

Brain damage predisposes a person to perseveration and echolalia by altering the brain's neurotransmitters. Psychologically, perseveration is a compulsive act and it is perpetuated, at least in part, by the patient's obsessive need to maintain integrity of self. This is not to say that obsessive-compulsive personality disorder causes perseveration and echolalia in aphasia; the two simply share common characteristics. The verbal and graphic responses, incorrect though they may be, give the patient the appearance of normalcy. For the patient, an inappropriate response is better than no response; he or she does not want to feel or appear communicatively impotent.

Perseveration and echolalia can have significant negative effects on speech and language rehabilitation by reducing the mental flexibility necessary for learning and adapting to the disability. It can also result in prolonged negative mental sets of anxiety, depression, hopelessness, and helplessness. Early initiation of treatment for patients with aphasia, especially for those with the tendency to perseverate, can counter habitual, perseverative negative thoughts which may be adopted by the patient without proper early intervention. By giving the patient abundant praise, support, and positive statements about his or her condition, the patient can avoid these negative thoughts about his or her disability.

The treatment of perseveration and echolalia involves creating mental flexibility in the patient, and can be incorporated into most aphasia therapies. The objective is for the patient to develop a flexible mental set during the therapies, and to improve his or her abilities to shift more rapidly and easily from one thought to another. Instruction and encouragement are given to motivate the patient, and verbal rewards are provided, not simply for the correct responses, but for the patient attempting to shift from one mental set and behavior to another.

Case Studies, Illustrations, and Examples: Perseveration and Echolalia

The patient's aphasia was caused by a large, dense stroke and rendered her unable to functionally express herself through speech and writing. Typically, when she would attempt to express herself verbally, the output would be something like this: "I want, want, want, I want, want … " The perseveration also manifested itself in echolalia. For example, when the clinician asked: "How are you today?" Her response was the last word she heard, "Today." Similarly, when the patient was asked if she wanted milk or juice, the reply was automatically juice, when in fact, she reached for the milk. About 90% of her output was echolalic repetitions of the last word she heard. The patient's writing was similarly perseverative with only the first letter of her name being legible, and the remaining writing meaningless markings on the paper gradually trailing off to a straight line. The patient was aware of her communication output, and she was frustrated by it.

Turn-taking counting, and other shared serial exercises, were helpful in reducing and controlling the perseveration and echolalia. During turn-taking counting exercises, the clinician would say, "One," and the patient encouraged to produce the next number in the sequence: "Two." Then, the clinician followed-up on the next number, "Three," with the patient responding with, "Four," and so forth. The goal of the therapy was to help the patient relearn the ability to shift from one stimulus to the next, and to inhibit the tendency to utter the last word heard. Similar turn-taking serial activities include days of the week, months of the year, and the alphabet.

To help reduce the frustration of the perseveration and echolalia, the turn-taking counting and other shared serial activities were conducted as fun games where the patient was encouraged to break the perseverative tendencies. The goal of the therapy was to help the patient break perseverative and echolalic behaviors by encouraging and verbally praising attempts to properly complete the activities.

EMOTIONAL LABILITY

Emotional lability is the involuntary exaggerated emotionality seen in some patients with neurogenic communication disorders. Several terms are used to describe emotional lability: pseudobulbar emotional lability, inappropriate crying, pseudobulbar affect, pathological emotionality, uncontrolled emotional expression, and emotional incontinence. Bilateral brain damage predisposes the patient to emotional lability, and it occurs in several diseases and disorders including stroke, traumatic brain injury, Alzheimer's disease, and amyotrophic lateral sclerosis. In neurogenic communication disorders, emotional lability is often seen in spastic dysarthria and bilateral damage to the motor strips of the brain and associated corticobulbar tracts. Like perseveration, emotional lability is a facet of the broad personality trait dominant Negative Affectivity (American Psychiatric Association, 2013).

Cummings et al. (2006) propose "involuntary emotional expression disorder" be used as a unifying label for patients with emotional lability following neurological injury. Unfortunately, the label inaccurately suggests that the emotionality is completely involuntary when most patients can exercise some inhibitory control. The label also indicates that emotions are limited to expression when patients can experience emotions without expressing them. The conventional label, emotional lability, should be retained because it accurately addresses the notion of emotional instability without unnecessarily limiting its parameters. "Lability" simply suggests "unstable" and "nonfixed," it does not address etiology, and it is commonly used to describe other medical conditions such as wide blood pressure fluctuations.

Although the research is unequivocal that brain damage predisposes patients to emotional lability, there is controversy concerning whether patients have true emotions associated with the acts of uncontrolled crying. Some authorities describe emotional lability as pathological emotionality without the authentic emotions linked to the stimuli that prompt the outbursts. Other authorities suggest that while involuntary emotional expressions occur in excess, most patients have normal underlying affect.

Regardless of the terms used to describe involuntary emotions occurring in neurological diseases and disorders, it should be noted that emotional lability is exaggerated and not inappropriate emotionality. Stimuli prompt the uncontrolled exaggerated emotional reactions, and patients have lowered emotional thresholds for expression. Certainly, the emotions are excessive, and usually involve crying because of the negativity associated with the patient's predicament. To propose that the crying behavior in these patients is "inappropriate" rather than "exaggerated" diminishes the patient's psychological response to his or her neurogenic communication disorders. In addition, assuming that all emotional reactions by the patient are pathological and inappropriate can create conditions where important quality-of-life issues for the patient are intellectualized and dismissed by health care professionals.

The triggers for emotional lability are similar to the stimuli causing emotional responses in normal people. The patient's thoughts, certain situations, and highly charged words can setoff bouts of emotional lability. Negative thoughts, particularly about the patient's predicament, can cause crying and many depressed patients are more likely to exhibit emotional lability. Excessive crying can alert health care professionals to a patient's underlying clinical depression. Situational triggers for emotional lability include visits by family and friends and frustrating therapeutic exercises. Gainotti (1989) suggested that emotional lability is a manifestation of a catastrophic reaction, a type of anxiety attack, in patients prone to crying. In therapeutic activities and conversations with the emotionally labile patient, certain words can prompt crying. Highly charged and emotional terms such as "nursing home," "stroke," and names of loved ones can stimulate exaggerated emotionality in some patients.

For patients with severe and prolonged bouts of emotional lability medication may be necessary to treat it successfully. Physicians may prescribe antidepressants or other medications to reduce or eliminate the patient's underlying negativity and anxiety. In a study by Scoppetta, Di Gennaro, and Scoppetta (2005), a selective serotonin reuptake inhibitor (SSRI), a type of antidepressant, was found to prevent emotional lability. However, even in these patients, therapeutic intervention should precede or accompany pharmacological treatment. Emotional lability during speech can significantly reduce intelligibility.

The "Three P" therapy for emotional lability, addressing the predisposing, precipitating, and perpetuating factors, can easily be incorporated into therapy for patients with communication disorders and reduce the frequency and duration of crying episodes. While brain damage is the primary predisposing factor in emotional lability, other factors make a patient more susceptible to excessive crying. Negative sleeping habits, lack of exercise, poor diet, and stress can exacerbate emotional lability in many patients. To reduce the predisposing factors in emotional lability, the patient should get plenty of sleep, exercise regularly, have a good diet, and keep stress at a minimum. Additionally, there is a natural reduction in the predisposing factors for emotional lability because of spontaneous recovery that occurs in most patients with aphasia except those with severe global involvement.

The second aspect of the therapeutic management of emotional lability concerns the precipitants, or triggers, that set off bouts of exaggerated crying. As discussed previously, thoughts, situations, and highly charged words can trigger excessive crying. Early post onset, attempts should be made to avoid as many situations and conversational triggers as possible. If possible, the patient should be counseled to redirect his or her thoughts to positive ones and away from negativity. As the patient regains emotional stability, he or she can gradually and systematically be exposed to the precipitating factors.

Perpetuating factors of emotional lability involve aspects of the behavior that cause continuation of the excessive crying. Redirection of the patient's attention can reduce the length and severity of bouts of emotional lability. Patients can be instructed to direct their attention to pleasant thoughts and positive images during episodes of emotional lability to reduce the duration and severity of the episodes.

The "Three P" therapy for emotional lability reduces or eliminates predisposing, precipitating, and perpetuating factors. It can be an effective treatment for patients with mild to moderate emotional lability. For patients with severe and prolonged emotional lability, it can be used in conjunction with medications to help patients with aphasia and other related disorders regain emotional stability.

Case Studies, Illustrations, and Examples: Emotional Lability

Christine, a woman in her mid-60s, suffered a stroke causing mild predominantly expressive aphasia and spastic dysarthria. She spent two weeks in a rehabilitation unit of a regional hospital and after discharge, she was seen as an outpatient twice weekly. The aphasic word-finding problems improved spontaneously as a result of therapies, which included rapid naming exercises and sentence completion tasks. The goal of the dysarthria treatment included improving voice quality, speech precision, and intelligibility. A serious concomitant of the aphasia and dysarthria was severe emotional lability, which interfered with the therapies, reduced her speech intelligibility, and was distressing to the patient and her husband.

Although emotional lability can include laughing, Christine primarily displayed crying behaviors. The crying behaviors were frequent, occurring ten or more times during a session, lengthy in duration, and severe in their manifestations. The incidences of crying behaviors lasted for several minutes. The precipitants of the bouts of emotional lability included stimulus words used in therapy and emotionally-charged situations.

Christine was highly motivated during rapid naming exercises and sentence completion tasks and participated in them enthusiastically. However, the therapies were frequently disrupted by the bouts of crying emotional lability precipitated by emotionally-charged words such as nursing home, doctor, nurse, body parts, and the names of grandchildren and other family members. For the patient, these words stimulated emotional lability because they prompted thoughts about her stroke, disabilities, and related unwanted changes in her life. Emotionally-charged situations precipitating emotional lability included visits by her husband, grandchildren, other family members, doctors, nurses, and therapists.

To address the emotional lability, emotionally-charged stimulus words were avoided. During the bouts of crying, the patient was encouraged to concentrate on positive or neutral visual imagery such as office pictures, jewelry, clothing, and pleasant window views. Over time, Christine's emotional lability decreased in frequency, duration, and severity due to spontaneous recovery, therapies, and antidepressants prescribed by her attending physician.

CATASTROPHIC REACTIONS

Anxiety disorders include panic attacks, phobias, acute stress disorders, generalized anxiety disorders, post-traumatic stress syndrome, and obsessive-compulsive disorders. A catastrophic reaction is one manifestation of a panic attack occurring in some patients with aphasia. According to the American Psychiatric Association (2013), patients with catastrophic reactions do not meet the clinical requirements of panic disorders if the panic attacks are judged to be a direct result of another medical condition.

The catastrophic reaction usually occurs when the patient is confronted with too much stimuli and faced with the likelihood of failure. At the core of the catastrophic reaction is the patient's loss of a sense of mental and physical integrity and communicative impotence. A catastrophic reaction may occur during speech and language therapy when too much is required of the patient and communicative failure is likely. Temporal urgency, the need to respond quickly, also may trigger a catastrophic reaction. Research shows that catastrophic reactions are more likely to occur in patients with damage in and around Broca's area and the resulting non-fluent speech output (Carota et al., 2001). There may also be an association between post stroke depression and the occurrences of catastrophic reactions since anxiety is often a component in depression and non-fluent aphasia is frustrating. Salas (2012) suggests that people experiencing catastrophic reactions may look for significant others to regulate themselves from the outside. Shehata, Mistikawi, Risha, and Hassan (2015) note that depression and anxiety are more prominent among patients with aphasia than in stroke patients without aphasia.

Jon Eisenson (1984) examined the catastrophic reaction in aphasic patients and considered it a psychobiological breakdown. The patient's panic is accompanied by physiological reactions such as increased blood pressure, muscular hypertension, sweating, and dry mouth. In extreme catastrophic reactions, a patient may strikeout physically and verbally, cry, and even lose consciousness. At the core of the physiological reactions in the catastrophic reaction is the fight or flight response. Physiologically, the patient prepares to flee or fight the perceived threat, and the human alarm system is triggered. While excessive therapeutic stimuli may prompt a catastrophic reaction, too much visual clutter and ambient noise may also trigger one.

Prevention is the best treatment for catastrophic reactions. Unfortunately, it may take one or more occurrences of observable catastrophic reactions before the clinician is aware that a patient is prone to them. When the patient is experiencing a catastrophic reaction, the clinician should provide immediate reduction in the stimuli and provide an avenue for him or her to escape such as leaving the room or closing eyes and resting. The clinician can also provide soothing, comforting, and calming statements. Katz (2000) suggests a key parameter in treating the catastrophic reaction is addressing environmental factors. Relaxation training may also be helpful in patients with the communicative abilities to benefit from it.

Case Studies, Illustrations, and Examples: Catastrophic Reactions

The experienced clinician knows lunchtime can be an excellent time to conduct aphasia therapy. Eating activities and food items provide many practical language stimuli for naming, recall, and sentence expansion therapies. For example, words such as the names of utensils and the color of food are stimuli having practical relevance for the patient. The clinician knows that stimuli for aphasia therapy should begin with egocentric concepts, such as names of body parts, clothing, family and friends, and expand outwardly to less self-centered stimuli. Of course, doing therapy at lunchtime requires the patient's permission which occurred with this individual.

During the lunchtime therapy, the patient was responding normally. As the complexity of the drills and exercises increased, she began to show signs of frustration. The patient turned her head rapidly from side-to-side and closed her eyes. There was also an increasing amount of noise in the dining room. Then, suddenly, the patient pushed the tray of food onto the lap of the clinician, spilling the contents. She made repeated attempts to pushed herself away from the table. This catastrophic reaction appeared to come out-of-the blue. Later, upon reflection, the clinician recognized that she did not appreciate the subtle indications of the impending anxiety reaction.

The increase in fidgeting, head turning, and eye-closing behaviors were all indications of the impending catastrophic reaction. These basic avoidance and escape behaviors increased in frequency as the complexity of the drills increased. The most significant precipitator of her catastrophic reaction was the presence of temporal urgency, and the pressure to respond quickly.

The clinician remembered a lecture on catastrophic reactions where the professor remarked that the first occurrences of these anxiety attacks are often unforeseeable and cannot be avoided. However, after the patient has shown a tendency for catastrophic reactions, it is the clinician's responsibility to control the environment in order to prevent future ones. The professor stated: "The clinician is not to blame for the first catastrophic reaction; however, he or she is at least partially responsible for subsequent ones." Accordingly, lunchtime therapies were discontinued and the patient was seen in her room or in a quiet therapy suite. The therapies were done in a more relaxed manner attempting to eliminate even the perception of temporal urgency. Care was taken to make the patient's room orderly and visitors were kept to a minimum. The patient's family and friends were counseled in the strategies to prevent catastrophic reactions. Additionally, during the weekly rehabilitation meeting, her case was discussed and the attending physician prescribed an antidepressant that reduces anxiety.

ORGANIC DEPRESSION-ANXIETY DISORDER

As discussed previously, patients with aphasia are predisposed to depression and anxiety. Upwards of 70% of people with predominantly expressive aphasia will experience depression-anxiety that is long lasting. Accurate incident and prevalence figures for depression and anxiety in patients with severe neurogenic communication disorders is unavailable due to the inability to get meaningful reports about their mental and emotional states. This is particularly true for global aphasic patients.

The depression-anxiety disorder seen in many patients with aphasia can be reactive and a part of the grief response, primarily the result of a chemical imbalance caused by the brain injury, or a combination of both causal factors. People with anxiety disorders often have an underlying depression, and anxiety is a frequent symptom of clinical depression. Whereas reactive depression occurring in the grief response usually does not include significant anxiety, organic depression is often associated with "a feeling of impending doom." The angst felt by patients is combination of despair and anxiety. Many patients become preoccupied and anxious with their mental and body changes. Some patients may experience predominantly anxiety or predominantly depression in the spectrum of the organically-based depression-anxiety disorder. The predominance of one over the other may change over time. The anxiety component in depression-anxiety disorder may be based on the patient's concern about his or her depressive thoughts and unsuccessful attempts to avoid and escape them. In most patients, there is a loss of the "joie de vivre," the carefree "joy of life" and pleasure in day-to-day living. With severe or chronic depression-anxiety, clinicians should be alert to indications of suicide and take immediate and appropriate prevention measures. Upwards of 15% of depressed people die by suicide and the incidence is higher among the elderly. The most important sign of suicide ideation is a report or indication from the patient, or his or her family, that suicide is being considered.

When brain damage predisposes a patient to depression and anxiety, it primarily is a consequence of a neurochemical imbalance. In patients with aphasia, neurochemicals such as serotonin and dopamine, which are associated with "feelings of well-being," are out of balance for maintaining positive mood and emotion. Decreased serotonin, in particular, is linked to depression and anxiety disorders. Nevertheless, there is always a psychological component to persistent depression-anxiety. The high incidence and prevalence of depression and anxiety in expressive non-fluent aphasic persons may also be related to the frustrating nature of the communication disorder. There is a strong correlation and causal relationship between stress and depression-anxiety.

Counseling and antidepressant medication therapies are the two primary treatments for organic depression-anxiety. Unfortunately, for many patients with aphasia, counseling, the "talking cure," is contraindicated. While counseling is important in a comprehensive treatment for depression-anxiety disorder in people with normal communicative abilities, for many patients with aphasia, it is impractical because of the communication barrier. Patients with moderate to severe aphasia do not have the communication abilities to benefit from counseling. In addition, counseling with these patients may exacerbate their depression-anxiety because of the frustration they might experience in being unable to communicate about the important issues brought up during the counseling sessions.

There are several antidepressant medications that effectively combat severe and prolonged depression-anxiety. Additionally, some herbs and dietary supplements may also have a positive effect in improving general mood, and in reducing mild-to-moderate depression and anxiety. Exercise is also helpful in reducing depression and anxiety. While all drugs have side effects, most antidepressant medications, when prescribed appropriately by a physician, are free from serious ones. Unfortunately, most antidepressants take several days and even weeks to begin to combat the depression-anxiety. In addition, physicians may try several different types and dosages of antidepressant medications before finding the optimal regimen. Of course, physicians rely on feedback from the patient about the ongoing effects of the medication and this feedback is not available from many patients with aphasia. In these circumstances, clinicians can be valuable indirect sources of information about the patient's depression-anxiety and general mood. Especially with global aphasic patients, if there appears to be depression-anxiety, it is humane to recommend antidepressant medication therapy. Most antidepressant medications can be taken indefinitely with few serious side effects.

Case Studies, Illustrations, and Examples: Organic Depression-Anxiety Disorder

Raymond, a 66-year-old patient with stroke-induced severe aphasia, displayed several symptoms of depression and anxiety. Although Ray was unable to verbally communicate his depression and anxiety, his nonverbal behaviors clearly showed the severe mood disorder and high levels of anxiety. His facial and body expressions were those of a person clearly in the grips of depression and he experienced several catastrophic reactions since the stroke. Most importantly, his wife of 35 years reported that she sensed he was extremely depressed and anxious.

During the rehabilitation meeting, the occupational and physical therapists reported Ray was depressed and getting more so. Several nurses who had frequent contact with the patient also reported indications of depression such as his reluctance to get out of bed in the mornings, avoidance of family and friends, loss of appetite, weight loss, and overall lethargy. At the conclusion of the rehabilitation meeting, Ray's physician said she would start him on an antidepressant that also countered anxiety. She noted that it would take about two weeks for the medication to fully address the depression and anxiety.

In aphasia therapy, the clinician engaged him in drills, counseling, and exercises thought to help combat depression and anxiety. A routine was established where the patient was awakened at the same time each day, therapies held at regular times, and meals provided in the dining room rather than bed. The patient was dressed in comfortable clothing, and the aphasia therapies were held in a bright solarium rather than in the therapy suite. Praise was given to Ray for attempting the therapies and even for small gains in communication abilities. Nurturing and self-esteem statements were frequently made such as "You are doing a great job," "You are OK," "You are improving," and "It's going to be all right." The clinician allowed and even encouraged a wide range of emotional expressions. On several occasions, Ray's wife participated in the therapies and was encouraged to be positive and supportive.

Within several days, the patient's mood appeared to gradually improve, and after about a week, the antidepressant appeared to produce positive results. There were no further occurrences of catastrophic reactions. After several weeks in the rehabilitation unit of the hospital, it was determined that Ray was globally aphasic and not likely to benefit significantly from continued aphasia therapies. The family was given educational material about global aphasia and activities they could engage in to help improve communication with him. Ray clearly benefitted from the antidepressant and continued with it for the remainder of his life.

ANOSOGNOSIA

In aphasia, anosognosia is the denial or lack of insight of disease or disability in people with brain injury. Denial is primarily a perceptual defense mechanism where the person blocks the reality of the situation from his or her conscious awareness (Tanner, 2012). The denial may be complete with the patient refusing to perceive or accept the totality of the disease or disability (Tanner and Gerstenberger, 1996). For example, a patient may not accept that a disordered limb is part of his body. Short-lived denial of hemiplegia occurs in more than half of patients with damage to the right hemisphere immediately after a stroke (Cutting, 1978). Carlat (1999) observed that extreme denial can be indicative of psychotic thought processes. Benson and Ardila (1996) noted that a patient with anosognosia may not see his or her disability in the proper perspective.

Some authorities limit the definition of anosognosia to "lack of awareness" of a disease or disability (American Psychiatric Association, 2013; Davis, 2007). However, active denial often co-occurs with lack of awareness especially in patients with visual neglect. In addition, insufficient information about the nature and course of an illness or disability may simply cause lack of awareness.

Anosognosia may occur with all neurogenic communication disorders, but it plays an important role in fluent jargon aphasia associated with damage to the Wernicke's area and adjacent sites and tracts of the left temporal-parietal lobes. In their classic articles, Weinstein and Puig-Antich (1974) and Weinstein et al. (1966) considered the denial of disability as partially responsible for the persistent jargon in Wernicke's aphasia patients. In some fluent jargon aphasic patients, the meaningless speech is persistently produced when functional communication is obviously not taking place. For example, a fluent jargon patient may utter a series of meaningless statements to a listener in an apparent attempt to obtain some good or service. There is clearly an attempt to express something important and meaningful. However, because the fluent jargon is incomprehensible to the listener, there is no consummation of the communicative act and consequently, no speaker satisfaction. Due to anosognosia, many fluent jargon aphasic patients continue to engage in meaningless speech acts even though it is apparent that functional communication does not take place.

Fluent jargon aphasic patients rarely pause for acknowledgment, or engage in turn-taking in conversations (Owens, Metz, and Haas, 2000). Many people with aphasia also act as if their jargon is perfectly normal, and if the listener would try harder to understand it, meaningful communication would take place. They are often irritated and angry with the listener's inability to understand their "perfectly normal" speech. A normal speaker would eventually see the futility of the fluent jargon for meaningful communication, and stop speaking altogether because of the listener's inability to understand. The anger and irritation at the listener's inability to comprehend their fluent jargon is partially a result of the psychological defense mechanism of projection. Projection is attributing one's intolerable wishes, thoughts, motivations, and feelings to another person.

The question may be asked, "Does fluent jargon have psychological meaning for the patient?" Of course, it is impossible to generalize accurately about the meaningless expressions produced by all aphasic patients. However, several possibilities exist for the psychological implications of jargon that go beyond denial and projection. First, fluent jargon may simply be a result of defective speech monitoring by the patient. Due to the receptive language disorder, the patient may be unable to accurately monitor his or her output. Consequently, the patient is not cognizant of the meaninglessness of the jargon and is essentially unaware that he or she is speaking abnormally. In effect, the patient perceives himself or herself as normal and others as abnormal. Second, psychologically, the jargon of the aphasic patient may be an attempt to maintain the integrity of self and the appearance of normal mental functions. By producing speech, albeit abnormal jargon, the patient maintains the illusion of normalcy, and it is psychologically meaningful for his or her continuity of self. Third, the fluent jargon aphasic patient may be producing jargon because of damaged semantic processing, and the output reflects his or her inner speech. The meaningless words and statements are meaningful to the patient and reflective of her or his cognitive processing. In this sense, it is a form of idioglossia, a private, distinctive language induced by brain damage.

The treatment of anosognosia involves gradual and systematic confrontation of the disease's or disability's manifestations and symptoms. This confrontation is done in a highly supportive and positive environment. If possible, the patient's family and friends should be present to offer support and encouragement. Never should the patient be brutally confronted with the reality of the disease or disability. Denial of disability serves as an important buffer to psychological pain. The patient's denial should be gradually reduced or eliminated with support and encouragement. It should be remembered that although brain damage predisposes the patient to anosognosia, there is always a psychological consequence that goes beyond the neurological issues.

Case Studies, Illustrations, and Examples: Anosognosia

Roy, a middle-aged male, was involved in a barroom brawl, and incurred a blunt force traumatic brain injury resulting in jargon aphasia. He was found unconscious in the parking lot of the bar and apparently had no recollection of the assault. He was initially seen in the acute care wing of the regional hospital, and was transferred to the rehabilitation center for intensive aphasia therapy.

Roy made few gains in his expressive and receptive language abilities and was generally unresponsive in therapy. He displayed a pleasant demeanor but would become agitated when confronted with corrections to his speech or given directional commands. He denied the communication disorder and became angry when the clinician would repeat his jargon. When asked to follow directional commands, Roy simply turned away from the table and refused to engage in therapy. A typical jargon utterance produced by the patient was "It all depends on the acrylic, thus far." He projected the attitude that his utterances were completely comprehensible and listeners should try harder to understand his "normal" speech.

A psychiatrist recommended that Roy be video recorded during aphasia therapy. He suggested having Roy watch the video recording would help him overcome his anosognosia and increase his responsiveness to therapy. After a 30 minute session was recorded, Roy was brought to a conference room to observe it. At first, the patient was cooperative and took an interest in the video. After several minutes, however, he became agitated and tried to leave the room. After he calmed down, Roy clearly, albeit with jargon speech, communicated: "The patient in the video did not have a communication disorder, and even if he did, he was not the person on the video."

Unfortunately, Roy never completely ceased the denial and projection, and although his comprehension improved, much of his jargon remained. Several years later, the clinician met the patient at a shopping mall and he responded to the question: "How are you doing?" with "It all depends on the acrylic, thus far."

HOMONYMOUS HEMIANOPSIA AND VISUAL NEGLECT

Homonymous hemianopsia is a type of cortical or perceptual blindness, which includes the loss of vision in one half of the same visual fields of both eyes. Visual neglect, which may occur with or without homonymous hemianopsia, involves the patient's inability and unwillingness to attend to one side of his or her body and environment. A patient with homonymous hemianopsia and visual neglect is sometimes said to have lost "half of his or her world." Brinbaum, Hackley, and Johnson (2015) observe that although patients with homonymous hemianopsia do not consciously see vision in the blind hemifield, there is evidence of a "blindsight" phenomenon in such patients. The blindsight phenomenon is the ability to detect objects without conscious awareness of being able to see them.

When a patient with aphasia has visual field disturbances, she or he may also have accompanying visual neglect. Severe visual field disturbance can affect reading, writing, and naming. Due to the patient's refusal or inability to cross midline during reading, he or she will only read one side of a page with a consequent reduction in reading comprehension. She or he will only read to the midline of the page. When writing, the patient will not write beyond the midline of a page. Similarly, when naming objects in the environment or in an array during testing, the patient will be compromised due to the visual field disturbances. In addition, some patients with homonymous hemianopsia and visual neglect will only consume food on one side of a plate, shave or apply makeup to one side of the face, and only attend to conversations occurring on one side of a room. According to Culbertson and Tanner (2015), in the case of hemianopsia, if opposite halves of the visual field are involved for each eye, the hemianopsia is heteronymous.

Homonymous hemianopsia and visual neglect are the result of central nervous system damage, often caused by stroke, neoplasms (tumors), or traumatic brain injury, and both disorders also have a strong psychological component. Psychologically, a partial explanation for the patient neglecting one side of the visual word is that unwanted physical changes have occurred on the affected side of his or her body. The hemiplegia threatens the patient's integrity of self and sense of wholeness. The visual neglect is partially a consequence of the coping style, and psychological defense of avoidance. By avoiding the negatively affected side of his or her world, the patient is partially and temporarily protected from anxiety and negative emotions.

The treatment for homonymous hemianopsia involves gradual and systematic therapies designed to have the patient confront his or her affected side and to cross midline. These therapies can occur during conversations, reading, writing, and object naming exercises held in the patient's room. If the patient also has dysphagia, a swallowing disorder, crossing midline during eating can also be a goal of therapy. Attempts by the patient to confront the negativity associated with the disordered side of his or her world should be encouraged in a positive and accepting environment, and each attempt to cross midline immediately praised and rewarded.

Case Studies, Illustrations, and Examples: Homonymous Hemianopsia and Visual Neglect

Mrs. Ruth Wannamaker, a 65-year-old woman, suffered an occlusion of the posterior cerebral artery and subsequent damage to the left occipital lobe. She presented with right homonymous hemianopsia and visual neglect. During testing, she would not identify objects placed in her right visual field. She would not acknowledge room objects on the right side of her hospital room. When conversing with people, she would track them as they moved from the left to the right in her visual field, but abruptly stop as they crossed visual midline. Interestingly, when talking to the examiner, even though she could normally hear the speech, she would not acknowledge the speaker when he moved into her right visual field. When applying makeup, she typically would only do so on the left side of her face.

Initially, Mrs. Wannamaker was prescribed special prism glasses to assist her vision but she rejected them; she found them confusing and anxiety-provoking. During reading exercises, she was encouraged to cross the midline of the page by turning her head to accommodate the visual field cut. Gradually, she learned to partially cross midline by having the clinician praise each attempt to do so. Similar therapies were provided to get the patient to cross midline during conversations as the speaker walked from one side of the room to another. In addition, the television in her room was placed on the right side of her visual field.

A therapy that was particularly helpful involved pushing the patient in her wheelchair down a vacant hallway and seeking objects placed in her defective visual field. Each object was shown to her in advance and placed on the floor, wall, or on tables in the hall. The goal was to find them by turning her head to accommodate the visual field cut and to confront and address the visual neglect. This therapy also helped the patient avoid hitting objects, and consequently improved her mobility.

EUPHORIA

Euphoria, an elevated mood and heightened sense of well-being, occurs in normal people, but also occurs from anoxia. For example, in flight training, pilots are taught that a sense of euphoria is an indication of oxygen deprivation at high altitudes, and that oxygen masks are required.

According to Craig and Cummings (1995), euphoria can be a chronic condition in fluent jargon aphasic patients. In normal people, euphoric episodes result from intensely exciting and pleasurable experiences, such as those involving love, sex, athletic achievements, religious conversions, and other experiences. It is interesting to note that in certain religious ceremonies where participants report euphoria, they often talk in "tongues," which has many similarities to aphasic jargon.

Denial may also result in euphoria. Denial, a radical perceptual defense to be discussed in Chapter 3, blocks the reality of the situation from the patient's consciousness leaving him or her with only positive thoughts and emotions. Ritchie (1961, pp. 35-36) observed:

> I heeded only the most obvious optimistic things that were said to me and for the rest I did not hear them or came to the conclusion that they were wrong. If I had allowed myself to be given a glimpse of the truth, I believe I would have gone out of my mind.

Should euphoria in the patient with aphasia be considered a negative rehabilitative and prognostic factor, and treated as a maladjustment to the disability? There are two issues regarding chronic euphoria in individuals with aphasia. First, the patient with euphoria has little anxiety about his disability and often seems unconcerned and even content with the predicament. Since the euphoric patient is unrealistic about his or her communication disorder, it can be considered a psychological maladjustment. The patient with persistent euphoria does not appreciate the reality of his or her situation. Although it appears that the euphoric patient has accepted his or her predicament, he or she is experiencing inappropriate and maladaptive emotions about it. Dissatisfaction with the status quo are primary motivators for patients to improve in rehabilitation, and euphoric patients lack this necessary ingredient to improve.

The second issue with euphoria in an aphasic patient involves the fact that there are few if any realistic treatments. It would seem inhumane and unkind to attempt to reduce or eliminate a patient's elevated mood and heightened sense of well-being. While the overriding goal may be to increase the patient's motivation and willingness to participate in rehabilitation, attempting to reduce or eliminate his or her euphoria is not a realistic, therapeutic objective. However, gradual confrontation of the patient to his or her disabilities and predicament in a supportive and positive environment may cause him or her to see the need to participate in rehabilitation.

Case Studies, Illustrations, and Examples: Euphoria

Duke, a 72-year-old former professor, suffered a traumatic brain injury resulting from an automobile accident. In addition to aphasia, apparent post-traumatic psychosis, disorientation, and dysarthria, he displayed an elevated mood. The elevated mood was associated with hallucinations and delusions involving the presence of his long-deceased father and mother. He reported their presence was comforting and resulted in "blissful" feelings.

Duke received reality orientation therapy, and unfortunately, the euphoria prohibited him benefitting from it. In reality orientation therapy, everyone in the hospital in contact with the patient would provide him with information regarding his condition, location, date and time, names of family members, and so forth. Pictures of family members, home, car, pets, and other important people and things in his life were prominently displayed on the hospital walls, and each visitor would remind him of them.

During the weekly rehabilitation meeting, members of the team reported that Duke was too euphoric to benefit significantly from the reality orientation and other rehabilitation therapies. The occupational therapist noted that Duke would not attend to many activities of daily living and simply sat contented in his chair. The speech-language pathologists reported the patient would not attend to aphasia, dysarthria, and reality orientation therapies, and appeared unconcerned about his inability to meaningfully communicate. Nursing, physical therapy, and neuropsychology also noted his euphoria and indifference.

Due to Duke's euphoria and indifference, it was determined that his ability to profit from many of the rehabilitation services was unlikely. He was discharged from the rehabilitation wing of the hospital and only certain physical therapies, where patient active participation was not required, were continued. The rehabilitation team agreed to monitor his status and they would resume intensive rehabilitation when the euphoria subsided.

TABLE 2-2

HYPERFUNCTIONAL AND HYPOFUNCTIONAL BEHAVIOR PATTERNS IN TRAUMATIC BRAIN INJURY

HYPERFUNCTIONAL BEHAVIOR PATTERNS	HYPOFUNCTIONAL BEHAVIOR PATTERNS
Hypersexuality	Hyposexuality
Aggressiveness	Apathy
Mood Swings	Flat affect
Impulsiveness	Reduced spontaneity
Increased socialness	Decreased socialness
Euphoria	Depression
Hyperattentive	Hypoattentive
Restlessness	Psychomotor retardation

MALADAPTIVE BEHAVIOR

Although all patients with aphasia may exhibit behavioral problems, Wernicke aphasia and traumatic brain injured patients often have significant behavioral issues affecting rehabilitation. Benson and Ardila (1996, p. 141) reported that behavioral problems in Wernicke aphasia patients are often dramatic:

> Wernicke aphasia patients often misinterpret their own problems and suspect that family members, friends, doctors, nursing staff, and others are the real cause of their comprehension difficulty. They accuse others of not listening carefully or of speaking in a code; this can lead to a suspicious, paranoid attitude producing an agitated, even dangerous behavior.

The behavioral problems in individuals with traumatic brain injuries can be divided into hyperfunctional and hypofunctional behavioral disorders (Table 2-2).

Hyperfunctional behavioral disorders include hypersexuality, aggressiveness, mood swings, impulsiveness, increased socialness, euphoria, increased attentiveness, and restlessness. Patients with hyperfunctional behavioral disorders appear unable to refrain and restrain excessive behaviors. Hypofunctional behavioral disorders include hyposexuality, apathy, reduced spontaneity, decreased socialness, depression, decreased attentiveness, and psychomotor retardation. Hypofunctional behavioral disorders often are seen in individuals with frontal lobe syndrome and can include significant response delay. Simpson, Sabaz, and Daher (2013) found that inappropriate sex talk was the most inappropriate sexual behavior in patients with traumatic brain injury followed by genital and nongenital touching behaviors, and exhibitionism or public masturbation. Patients with hypofunctional behavioral disturbances seem to lack energy, and have lost the will to engage in day-to-day activities. While all of the above behavioral disorders may occur in people without brain injury, neurological insult can predispose patients with aphasia to them.

Ylvisaker, Szekeres, and Feeney (2001) note that behavioral and psychosocial difficulties may be the result of a traumatic brain injury, but they are often complicated by preinjury challenges and postinjury adjustment problems.

Our work with several hundred adolescents and young adults with chronic school and work problems and general community reintegration difficulty suggests that behavioral and psychosocial themes are often at the core of these problems, although in most cases complex patterns of interaction exist between cognition and behavioral consequences of the injury. (Ylvisaker, Szekeres, and Feeney, 2001, p. 777)

Patients who make frequent commanding, ordering, and demanding statements may be feeling confused and disoriented, and their behaviors are attempts to take control of their lives.

Improvement of the patient's mental executive functioning (metacognition) is a primary long-term rehabilitation goal for people with traumatic brain injury. The rehabilitation team works cooperatively to manage the adjustment problems of the patient with particular emphasis on the risk factors associated with his or her discharge to home. The same primary long-term rehabilitation goal is applied to Wernicke aphasia patients predisposed to paranoid ideation or dangerous behaviors.

Case Studies, Illustrations, and Examples: Maladaptive Behavior

A 44-year-old male suffered a traumatic brain injury from an airplane crash resulting in several communication disorders. He was initially seen in the acute care wing of the hospital, and was transferred to the rehabilitation unit after about three weeks. He had significant retrograde amnesia, disorientation times four, and was hypersexual. He had an attentive wife who participated in therapies when possible.

This patient's hypersexuality was remarkable because of the frequency of his sexual comments and behaviors. Initially, virtually every statement he made to his wife and others were sexual in nature and understandably, his speech and behaviors were distressing to his wife. Even on the telephone, his speech was laced with vulgar words, propositions, and sexual innuendoes. His wife reported that he was premorbidly normal in regard to his sexuality, and his actions were out-of-character for him. She also noted that previously, he rarely used profanity.

During an elevator ride with his wife and an aide, the patient attempted to fondle the aide. His wife was aghast at his behavior and embarrassed. During a visit from a female acquaintance, the patient grasped her breast while making vulgar comments. On several occasions, the patient entered the hospital hall without clothing. He also frequently touched his genitals and attempted to masturbate in public.

Counseling was provided to the patient's wife and other visitors having contact with him. They were told that he was not responsible for his hypersexual behaviors, and though inappropriate, they were sometimes a temporary and necessary part of recovery from some traumatic brain injuries. In addition, it was explained that sexual drives are very powerful in most humans, and his loss of mental executive control allowed their free expression. The patient's wife was told that health care professionals often see these behaviors in traumatically brain injured patients and are accustomed to them.

Behavior modification was employed to combat the patient's inappropriate hypersexual behaviors. He was discouraged from engaging in them, but rarely punished for his actions. He was provided with verbal and institutional rewards for normal behaviors. Gradually, the frequency of inappropriate sexual behaviors decreased, and by the time he was discharged from the hospital, there were fewer of them. Interestingly, several months later when told of his actions, he had no recollection, nor did he acknowledge them. Table 2-3 lists, describes, and provides the psycho-organic maladaptive reactions in neurogenic communication disorders.

TABLE 2-3

PSYCHO-ORGANIC MALADAPTIVE REACTIONS IN NEUROGENIC COMMUNICATION DISORDERS

PSYCHOLOGICAL REACTION	DESCRIPTION	REHABILITATION OBJECTIVES
Emotional Lability	Involuntary, exaggerated emotionality	Reduce or eliminate the predisposing, precipitating, and perpetuating factors
Catastrophic Reaction	Psychological breakdown; panic attack	Prevention and minimization
Perseveration	Inappropriate continuation of an act and mental set	Mental flexibility
Organic Depression-Anxiety Disorder	Organically-based depression and anxiety	Environmental manipulation, counseling, antidepressant medication
Anosognosia	Denial of disease or disability	Gradual and systematic confrontation of the disease or disability manifestations and symptoms
Homonymous Hemianopsia and Visual Neglect	Cortical or perceptual blindness	Gradual and systematic exercises to confront the affected side and cross midline
Euphoria	Elevated mood and heightened sense of well-being	Gradual confrontation of the patient to his or her disabilities and predicament
Maladaptive Behavior	Hyperfunctional and hypofunctional behavior disorders; paranoia	Improvement of mental executive functioning (metacognition)

CHAPTER SUMMARY

Some patients with aphasia and related disorders are predisposed to psychological dysfunction and maladaptive behaviors because of the nature, type, and location of the brain injury. Exaggerated emotionality, catastrophic reactions, and perseveration occur in some patients resulting in excessive crying, panic attacks, and the impaired ability to shift mentally. Many patients with aphasia also suffer from depression and anxiety that are long lasting. Brain damage can also predispose a patient to denial of disability and visual neglect. Wernicke aphasia and traumatic brain injured patients may also have psycho-organically based maladaptive behaviors.

REFERENCES

American Psychiatric Association. (2013). *Diagnostic and statistical manual of mental disorders* (5th ed.). Arlington, VA: American Psychiatric Association.

Benson, F. D., and Ardila, A. (1996). *Aphasia: A clinical perspective.* New York, NY: Oxford University Press.

Black, F. (1975). Unilateral brain lesions and MMPI performance: A preliminary study. *Perceptual and Motor Skills,* 40(1), 87-93.

Brinbaum, F., Hackley, S., and Johnson, L. (2015). Enhancing visual performance in individuals with cortical visual impairment (homonymous hemianopsia): Tapping into blindsight. *Journal of Medical Hypotheses and Ideas, 9*(2), Supplement: S8-S13.

Carlat, D. (1999). *The psychiatric interview.* Philadelphia, PA: Lippincott, Williams & Wilkins.

Carota, A., Rossetti, A., Karapanayiotides, T., and Bogousslavsky, J. (2001). Catastrophic reaction in acute stroke: A reflex behavior in aphasic patients. *Neurology, 57*(10), 1902-1905.

Craig, A., and Cummings, J. (1995). Neuropsychiatric aspects of aphasia. In H. Kirshner (Ed.). *Handbook of neurological speech and language disorders* (pp. 483-498). New York, NY: Marcel Dekker, Inc.

Culbertson, W., and Tanner, D. (2015). *The Anatomy and Physiology of Speech and Swallowing.* Dubuque, IA: Kendall-Hunt.

Cummings, J. L., Arciniegas, D. B., Brooks, B. R., Herndon, R. M., Lauterbach, E. C., Pioro, E. P., Robinson, R. G., Scharre, D. W., Schiffer, R. B., and Weintraub, D. (2006). Defining and diagnosing involuntary emotional expression disorder. *CNS Spectrums, 11*(6), 1-7.

Cutting, J. (1978). Study of anosognosia. *Journal of Neurology, Neurosurgery and Psychiatry, 41*(6), 548-555.

Davis, G. A. (2007). *Aphasiology: Disorders and clinical practice* (2nd ed.). Boston, MA: Pearson, Allyn and Bacon.

Eisenson, J. (1984). *Adult aphasia,* (2nd ed.). Englewood Cliffs, NJ: Prentice-Hall.

Gainotti, G. (1972). Emotional behavior and hemisphere side of the lesion. *Cortex, 8*(1), 41-55.

Gainotti, G. (1989). The meaning of emotional disturbances resulting from unilateral brain injury. In G. Gainotti, & C. Caltagirone (Eds.), *Emotions and the dual brain.* New York, NY: Springer-Verlag.

Gasparini, W., Satz, P., Heilman, K., and Coolidge, F. (1978). Hemispheric asymmetries of affective processing as determined by the Minnesota Multiphasic Personality Inventory. *Journal of Neurology, Neurosurgery and Psychiatry, 41*(5), 470-473.

Gordon, W., Hibbard, M., Egelko, S., and Diller, L. (1985). The multifaceted nature of the cognitive deficits following stroke: Unexpected findings. *Archives of Physical Medicine and Rehabilitation, 66,* 338.

Gordon, W., Hibbard, M., and Morganstein, S. (1996). Response to Tanner and Gerstenberger. In C. Code, & D. Muller (Eds.), *Forums in clinical aphasiology* (pp. 319-321). London, UK: Whurr.

Kaplan, E., Gallagher, R. E., and Glosser, G. (1998). Aphasia-related disorders. In M. Sarno (Ed.), *Acquired aphasia* (3rd ed., pp. 309-340). San Diego, CA: Academic Press.

Katz, I. R. (2000). Agitation, aggressive behavior, and catastrophic reaction. *International Psychogeriatrics, 12,* 119-123 Cambridge University Press.

Lipsey, J., Spencer, W., Rabins, P., and Robinson, R. (1986). Phenomenological comparison of poststroke depression and functional depression. *American Journal of Psychiatry, 143*(4), 527-529.

Morganstein, S., and Smith, M. (2001). Thematic language stimulation therapy. In R. Chapey (Ed.), *Language intervention strategies in aphasia and related neurogenic communication disorders* (4th ed.). Philadelphia, PA: Lippincott Williams & Wilkins.

Owens, R., Metz, D., and Haas, A. (2000). *Introduction to communication disorders.* Boston, MA: Allyn & Bacon.

Ritchie, D. (1961). *Stroke: A Study of recovery.* Garden City, NJ: Doubleday.

Robinson, R. (1986). Depression and stroke. *Psychiatric Annals, 17*(11), 731-740.

Robinson, R., and Benson, D. (1981). Depression in aphasic patients: Frequency, severity, and clinical-pathological correlations. *Brain and Language, 14,* 282-291.

Robinson, R., Boston, J., Starkstein, S., and Price, T. (1988). Comparison of mania and depression after brain injury: Causal factors. *American Journal of Psychiatry, 145*(2), 172-178.

Robinson, R., Lipsey, J., Bolla-Wilson, K., Bolduc, P., Pearlson, G., Rao, K., and Price, T. (1985). Mood disorders in left-handed stroke patients. *American Journal of Psychiatry, 142*(12), 1424-1429.

Sackeim, H., Greenberg, M., Weiman, A., Gur, R., Hungerbahler, J., and Geschwin, N. (1982). Hemispheric asymmetry in the expression of positive and negative emotions: Neurological evidence. *Archives of Neurology, 39,* 210-218.

Sackeim, H., and Weber, S. (1982). Functional brain asymmetry in the regulation of emotion: Implications for bodily manifestations of stress. In L. Goldberger, & S. Bernitz (Eds.), *Handbook of stress* (pp. 183-199). New York, NY: Macmillan.

Salas, C. (2012). Surviving catastrophic reactions after brain injury: The use of self-regulation and self-other regulation. *Neuropsychoanalysis, 14*(1), 77-92.

Sandson, J., and Albert, M. (1984). Varieties of perseveration. *Neuropsychologia, 22*(6), 715-32.

Scoppetta, M., Di Gennaro, G., and Scoppetta C. (2005). Selective serotonin reuptake inhibitors prevent emotional lability in healthy subjects. *European Review for Medical and Pharmacological Sciences,* (6), 343-348.

Shehata, G., Mistikawi, T., Risha, A., and Hassan, H. (2015). The effect of aphasia upon personality traits, depression and anxiety among stroke patients. *Journal of Affective Disorders 172,* 312-314.

Simpson, G., Sabaz, M., and Daher, M. (2013). Prevalence, clinical features, and correlates of inappropriate sexual behavior after traumatic brain injury: A multicenter study. *Journal of Head Trauma Rehabilitation, 28*(3), 202-210.

Smeltzer, D., Nasrallah, H., and Miller, S. (1994). Psychotic disorders. In J. Silver, S. Yudofsky, and R. Hales (Eds.), *Neuropsychiatry of traumatic brain injury.* Washington, DC: American Psychiatric Press.

Tanner, D. (2007). *The medical-legal and forensic aspects of communication disorders, voice prints, and speaker profiling.* Tucson, AZ: Lawyers and Judges Publishing Company.

Tanner, D. (2009). *The psychology of neurogenic communication disorders: A primer for health care professionals.* New York, NY: iUniverse.

Tanner, D. (2010). *Exploring the psychology, diagnosis, and treatment of neurogenic communication disorders.* New York, NY: iUniverse.

Tanner, D. (2012). Defense mechanisms and coping styles in aphasia. In R. Goldfarb (Ed). *Translational speech-language pathology and audiology: Essays in honor of Dr. Sadanand Singh.* San Diego, CA: Plural

Tanner, D., and Gerstenberger, D. (1996). Clinical forum 9: The grief model in aphasia. In C. Code, & D. Muller (Eds.), *Forums in clinical aphasiology,* (pp. 313-318). London, UK: Whurr.

Tardiff, K. (1997). Evaluation and treatment of violent patients. In D. Stoff, J. Breiling, and J.D. Maser (Eds.), *Handbook of antisocial behavior* (pp. 445-453). New York, NY: John Wiley & Sons.

Weinstein, E., Lyerly, O., Cole, M., and Ozer, M. (1966). Meaning in jargon aphasia. *Cortex, 2*(2), 165-187.

Weinstein, E., and Puig-Antich, J. (1974). Jargon and its analogues. *Cortex, 10*(1), 75-83.

Williams, W., Evans, J., and Fleminger, S. (2003). Neurorehabilitation and cognitive-behaviour therapy of anxiety disorders after brain injury: An overview and a case illustration of obsessive-compulsive disorder. *Neuropsychological Rehabilitation, 13*(1 & 2), 133-148.

Ylvisaker, M., Szekeres, S. F., and Feeney, T. (2001). Communication disorders associated with traumatic brain injury. In R. Chapey (Ed.), *Language intervention strategies in aphasia and related neurogenic communication disorders* (4th ed.). Philadelphia, PA: Lippincott Williams & Wilkins.

Psychology of Aphasia

Defense Mechanisms and Coping Styles

"Sometimes a cigar is just a cigar"

Sigmund Freud

CHAPTER PREVIEW

This chapter examines the role psychological defense mechanisms and coping styles play in the psychological adjustment to aphasia and other related disorders. Psychological threats are analyzed on the basis of whether they are stimulated by external or internal factors. Avoidance, ego restriction, physical escape, and autistic fantasy are discussed as ways people with aphasia may cope with threats of a predominantly external nature. Psychological defense mechanisms and coping styles available to language-deprived patients for threats of a predominantly internal nature are discussed. This includes denial, repression, psychological regression, passive-aggression, reaction formation, altruism, sublimation, substitution, displacement and projection, and dissociation. Psychological defense mechanisms and coping styles compromised by the loss of language are reviewed including rationalization and intellectualization, suppression, undoing, and humor.

DEFENSE MECHANISMS AND COPING STYLES

According to Porcerelli and Hibbard (2004, p. 466), Sigmund Freud (1856-1939) introduced the concept of defense mechanisms in 1894: "He conceptualized defenses as mental forces that opposed unacceptable ideas or feelings that, if acknowledged, would cause significant distress." Anna Freud (1895-1982), Sigmund Freud's daughter, continued his work regarding psychoanalysis and identified several defense mechanisms. While Sigmund Freud considered defense mechanisms primarily unconscious processes, there is a conscious organization to them. It is generally accepted

Tanner, D.C.
The Psychology of Aphasia: A Practical Guide for Health Care Professionals
(pp 53-79). © 2017 Taylor & Francis Group.

that while the mechanisms of psychological defenses are subconscious, their behaviors are conscious and observable. Halim and Sabri (2013) report a relationship between defense mechanisms and coping styles although they are dissimilar in terms of the cognitive operations involved.

Wallerstein (1999) noted that because defense mechanisms are theoretical abstractions, it is irrelevant whether they are conscious or subconscious. (In this text, "unconscious" refers to loss of consciousness because of brain injury, and "subconscious" refers to thought processes, drives, and emotions below the person's conscious awareness.) Wallerstein (1999) also noted that defense mechanisms are hypothetical constructs denoting the way the mind functions. While defense mechanisms and coping styles play an important explanatory role in contemporary mental health, there is controversy about their nature and adaptive values. Carlat (1999) first described defense mechanisms and coping styles as similar concepts; they are thoughts and behaviors used to reduce stress.

Defense mechanisms and coping styles are ways humans protect themselves from full awareness of distressing thoughts, feelings, drives, memories, situations, and ideas. Porcerelli, Thomas, Hibbard, and Cogan (1998) noted that the concept of ego defense mechanisms has stood the test of time, and provides important information about normal development, psychopathology, and adaptation. Today, the specific nature and manifestations of certain defense mechanisms and coping styles are controversial. The fact that people use them to contend with reality, protect themselves from anxiety, and to exclude disturbing thoughts from consciousness, is not controversial. Defense mechanisms and coping styles are important to individuals as a means to maintain self-esteem. Self-esteem is a personal judgement of worth based on a self-ideal, and derived from perceptions of self and the judgments of others.

Generally, psychological defense mechanisms and coping styles can be placed on a continuum of adaptability ranging from mature and adaptive to those that are immature, maladaptive, neurotic, and radical attempts to cope with stressors. Immature, maladaptive, neurotic, and radical psychological defense mechanisms and coping styles are used when stressors, and the individual's ability to cope with them, become overwhelming. Wallerstein (1999, p. 59) observed:

> Defenses or defensive behaviors can be viewed as complexly layered and, depending on whether the perspective is 'upward' syntonic and conscious or 'downward' toward the more archaic (infantile) and unconscious, can be seen to serve impulsive discharge pressures in relation to the higher psychic layerings or defensive avoidant needs in relation to the lower psychic layerings.

Unfortunately, in the psychology and psychiatric literature on psychological defense mechanisms and coping styles, there is no consensus on the nature and adjustment value of each psychological defense mechanism and coping style. In addition, the use of a certain psychological defense mechanism and coping style, and its productive contribution to mental health, is dependent on the nature of the stressor and how extensively and appropriately it is used. Even a mature defense mechanism and coping style can be maladaptive when used inappropriately.

DEFENSE MECHANISMS AND COPING STYLES IN APHASIA

Defense mechanisms and coping styles are important to understanding aphasia and related disorders for two reasons. First, defense mechanisms and coping styles play an important role in the psychological adaptation to disabilities. They affect the symptoms of neurogenic communication disorders and treatment efficacy. Second, in language-deprived aphasic patients, only nonverbal defense mechanisms may be available for coping and adjustment to the disability. Patients without language, global aphasics, have special adjustment challenges and issues not experienced by persons with normal intact language functions. Even in aphasic patients with partial language, the utilization of verbal defense mechanisms and coping styles may be impaired or less accessible (Tanner, 2003, 2012).

In the discussion that follows, several psychological defenses and coping styles will be reviewed relative to their application to patients with aphasia and the likelihood of being utilized by language-deprived people. It is acknowledged that some of the psychological defenses and coping styles discussed below are controversial concerning their definitions and adaptive value. However, it is necessary to review possible ways patients with aphasia may attempt to adjust to their disabilities and cope with the limitations caused by them.

PREDOMINANTLY EXTERNAL THREATS

Defense mechanisms and coping styles are patterned thoughts, feelings, drives, memories, and ideas that arise in response to perceived or real internal or external threats. They can be subconscious defense mechanisms and occur as an involuntary response, or they can be conscious coping styles. When the perceived threats and dangers are primarily prompted by an internal thought or memory, the defense mechanism and coping style depends on avoidance of this thought or memory. Perceived threats and dangers, primarily internal in nature, and the defense mechanisms and coping styles used to deal with them, are difficult to discover in many patients with aphasia because of communication impairments. When the perceived threats and dangers are prompted by external threats and dangers, the defense mechanisms and coping styles involve avoidance and physical escape from specific situations and environments. The primary defense mechanisms and coping styles used by patients with aphasia in dealing with external threats are: avoidance, ego restriction, physical escape, and autistic fantasy.

Avoidance

Avoidance is a basic and innate defense mechanism and coping style. When a person is confronted with unpleasantness, he or she can simply try to avoid it. It is often used when a person is confronted with an external threat, although avoidance of disturbing thoughts lies at the core of many defense mechanisms and coping styles. Avoidance is often used to deal with the potential of rejection and consequent threats to self-esteem. It also involves a tendency to circumvent cues, activities, and situations that remind the individual of stressful experiences (American Psychiatric Association, 2013).

There are two types of avoidance: postponement and refusal. In postponement, the avoiding person delays confronting the anxiety provoking situation, which provides temporary relief. The refusing person declines confronting the distressing and anxiety provoking stimulus, often after repeated postponements. The extreme use of avoidance creates the avoidant personality disorder: "These patients experience few positive reinforcers from self or others, are relentlessly vigilant and on guard, and are quick to distance themselves from anxious anticipation of life's painful and negatively reinforcing experiences" (Millon and Meagher, 2004, p. 109). As aforementioned, avoidance as a defense mechanism and coping style may be misunderstood and inappropriately addressed during evaluations and treatments in patients with aphasia.

In people with neurogenic communication disorders, there is much to avoid. Many patients must undergo painful therapies and invasive diagnostic procedures. The very nature of many therapies requires the patient to confront his or her disabilities, often with little time to prepare psychologically for that confrontation. This is particularly true concerning speech and language therapies because awareness of errors and monitoring of those errors are essential treatment objectives. Another major negative consequence of neurogenic communication disorders prompting the avoidance defense mechanism is confinement to a medical facility with new demands, routines, and often a near-total lack of privacy. There are also the costs of the medical care and the neurogenic communication disorder's implications on the patient's future employment and quality-of-life.

The use of avoidance as a defense mechanism and coping style should be understood, permitted, and in some cases, encouraged. When used appropriately and sparingly, this defense mechanism can provide necessary relief from the negativity and stresses associated with the neurogenic communication disorder. For many patients, attempts to postpone or refuse diagnostic procedures and treatments are adaptive ways of coping with the communication disorder, at least in the short-term.

Efforts should be taken to encourage the avoiding patient to participate fully in the rehabilitation program by providing support, counseling, and gradual confrontation with negative aspects of the neurogenic communication disorder. However, ultimately, it is the patient's prerogative to decide whether he or she participates in rehabilitation, when, and to what extent. While many patients with aphasia cannot express their rationale for using avoidance, this defense mechanism and coping style should be understood, tolerated, and respected. By doing so, health care professionals, family, and friends of the patient ultimately increase the likelihood that the patient will eventually be optimally motivated to participate in rehabilitation.

Avoidance is the simplest known defense mechanism and coping style and easily utilized by young children; avoidance does not require language to be effectively used. Consequently, language-deprived patients can avoid threatening and unpleasant situations and related thoughts by engaging in avoidance. When used sparingly, postponement and refusal can be adaptive ways of coping with the stressors associated with aphasia which deprive the patient of language. For global aphasic patients, the avoidance defense mechanism and coping style may be one of few ways of finding relief from the negativity and unpleasantness associated with this communication disorder.

Case Studies, Illustrations, and Examples: Avoidance

It is pleasant to be able to get around by yourself. You have learned to move from one place to another in the wheelchair. You must pull and push with your left foot, roll the wheel with your left hand, but you can get around. Freedom of independent movement is one of the few pleasures in your life. But the pleasant thoughts of freedom of movement are rapidly dampened by the approaching appointment time for occupational therapy. Although the resourceful occupational therapist amazes you with knowledge of alternatives, there are the frustrating attempts to move food from the plate to your mouth, difficulty putting on your clothes, and worst of all, the embarrassment of relearning the necessities of the bathroom. With all that has happened, you just want to be left alone.

You wheel the chair down the hall as fast as possible. You know the occupational therapy aide will soon be at your door, eager to transport you to the therapy room. Finally, you find the solarium and manage to get the wheelchair through the door just in time. Ah, safety. You won't have to suffer the indignities of occupational therapy. Today, at least, your mind and body can have a reprieve from negativity.

Ego Restriction

Anna Freud first identified the defense mechanism and coping style of ego restriction. In ego restriction, a type of avoidance, a person abandons an activity in response to anxiety. In the extreme, the individual voluntarily gives up an entire area of ego involvement rather than risk the possibility of not succeeding at it. The anxiety seen in ego restriction is based on threats to self-esteem.

The patient with aphasia knows he or she has suffered brain damage and this knowledge threatens his or her self-concept. The patient faces the reality that he or she cannot perform many day-to-day activities as well as he or she did previously. Additionally, the patient may be aware that others, including health care professionals, are examining, analyzing, and judging his or her behaviors and actions. Aphasia is fertile ground for questions regarding mental and physical competence.

An early aphasiologist, Joseph Wepman, noted that in all instances of brain damage, there appears to be some reduction in the person's self-esteem. Self-esteem is derived from perceptions of self and the judgments of others. Although the amount of reduction in self-esteem and the extent of the brain injury is not necessarily linear and does not have a one-to-one relationship, it is a positive one. With the obvious exceptions of patients who are euphoric or engage in persistent denial, the greater the brain injury, the more they appear to suffer from reductions in self-esteem. Aware patients appreciate that they have suffered brain damage, and thus are unlikely to have the abilities, thoughts, attitudes, and communication abilities they once possessed. The patient with aphasia must change his or her identity based on the realities of the new disabilities.

Patients with aphasia may display ego restriction in employment, family roles, social and recreation activities, and participation in rehabilitation. In employment, a patient may abandon an aspect of an occupation, or even an entire vocation, because of ego restriction. The patient's abandonment of an employment activity is not due to realistic inabilities to perform them due to the aphasia, it is a result of anxiety associated with the threats to self-esteem should he or she fail. He or she may also similarly abandon an important family function, such as taking a leadership role in purchasing matters. Ego restriction may be seen in social activities, especially those requiring extensive communication. In rehabilitation, a patient may abandon the role of a willing and motivated patient, not because he or she has a poor prognosis, but because the potential for failure provokes unacceptable levels of anxiety.

Case Studies, Illustrations, and Examples: Ego Restriction

Few things in life gave you more pleasure than the late-morning coffee-breaks with your friends. You loved gourmet coffee. Lattes, espressos, mochas, or other expensive coffee was a delight for the senses. You eagerly anticipated the smell, sight, taste, and the caffeine buzz the coffee provided. Added to the delight of the coffee was the conversation. You and your friends would sit in the corner of the airy coffee shop, admiring the pastoral paintings, watching customers, enjoying the fresh air, and having fervent discussions ranging from politics to grandchildren. The stroke changed all that.

Your speech is near-normal after weeks of rehabilitation, and your recall of the names of people and things have largely returned. You can make the sounds of speech relatively clear if you speak slowly and remember to exaggerate them. Oh sure, there is an abnormality to your speech, a sort of weird accent, but most people can understand you. You can make your thoughts known.

Your friends repeatedly invite you to return to the coffee shop. They sorely miss you, but you won't hear of it. You won't even entertain the thought of returning to the coffee shop. You have brain damage. You know you will have trouble getting to and from the coffee shop, ordering, and conversing. You won't risk the awful pangs of failure. You will stay home where it is safe and secure. No wheelchair ramps, no confused servers, no misunderstandings. Coffee-breaks with your friends are a thing of the past. They now are memories of better days, and you are perfectly content to let them go.

Physical Escape

Like avoidance, escape is an innate and basic defense mechanism and coping style providing immediate relief from anxiety. When avoidance is impractical or impossible, it may be necessary for a person physically to escape a negative or threatening situation thereby providing psychological relief. Anxiety is reduced when the person leaves. In patients with aphasia, the psychological need to physically escape from negative or threatening thoughts and situations may occur during evaluations and therapies. Patients with functional speech and language can report their need to escape a specific negative situation. They may say, "This is a stressful therapy, can we take a break?" or "Let's take a breather from this therapy and do something else now." Patients without functional speech and language may show their need to physically escape through fidgeting, agitation, and distraction behaviors.

Physical escape is observed in patients with aphasia when they are confronted with external threats, but like avoidance, the need to escape from disturbing thoughts lies at the core of many defense mechanisms and coping styles (Tanner, 2010, 2012). Jon Eisenson observed that a catastrophic reaction (See Chapter 2) is a psychobiological breakdown, which in the extreme, can result in the patient losing consciousness. Since the catastrophic reaction is based on the need to fight or flee from a perceived threat, a patient's loss of consciousness can be considered, at least on a psychological level, as the ultimate escape. By losing consciousness, the patient escapes from the external threat of the situation and the accompanying distressing thoughts.

As noted previously, patients with aphasia may disguise their reasons to escape from threatening therapeutic situations by feigning the need to go to the bathroom, wanting to return to their room for clothing, objects, or illness, and so on. Especially in patients with nonfunctional speech and language abilities, these disguised reasons for escaping from threatening therapeutic situations may only involve nonverbal indications of distress by the patient. Of course, this is not to say that all nonverbal requests by patients with nonfunctional speech and language abilities to stop a therapy and do something else are based on the escape psychological defense mechanism and coping style. However, escape from a threatening therapeutic situation should be considered, especially in patients with adjustment challenges. Like avoidance, escape should be understood, permitted, and sometimes encouraged.

Many patients with severe aphasia may be unable to verbalize the need to escape a threatening situation. Often, there are only nonverbal indications that he or she needs to escape, such as agitation, fidgeting, and distraction. When these indications are present, his or her wishes should be honored. Time out from demanding therapies and procedures should be provided to patients indicating escape needs. Where it is necessary to undergo procedures and therapies, the patient should be gradually exposed to them with ample opportunities to escape the negativity. She or he should be able to pause threatening procedures and therapies until she or he can mobilize the psychological resolve to undergo them.

Case Studies, Illustrations, and Examples: Physical Escape

Sometimes, you dread physical therapy. It hurts and forces you to deal with your defective arm. You cringe at the thought of being wheeled to the gym where it seems everyone watches your every movement, or lack thereof. The sling holding your spastic arm is taken away and strong, skilled hands pull, stretch, and try to increase its movement. Each movement sends flashes of pain down your back. Your stomach turns to knots, and the anxiety and pain is unbearable.

As the pain builds and the anxiety becomes too great, you try to find an escape. You utter a few words expressing your need to quit this painful and disturbing activity, but because of your communication disorder, the meaning is lost, or was never there. The physical therapist seems oblivious or indifferent to your plight. You can't stand it.

Finally, you gesture the need to go to the bathroom. You make urgent noises and point to the handicapped restroom. At last, the pain and the anxiety end and you are wheeled to safety. You do everything you can to burn time, and manage to spend the rest of the session in the rest room, free from the physical and psychological pain of your defective arm.

Autistic Fantasy

Autistic fantasy is a form of escape through excessive daydreaming and a symbolic way of meeting psychological needs. It is excessive fantasizing as a substitute for more appropriate action to deal with emotional conflicts. During fantasy escapes, the person retreats and withdraws into an imaginary world. Typical fantasy escapes include daydreaming about occupational, athletic, sexual, financial, family and social activities, and so forth.

Fantasy also can be embedded in the subconscious mind, and influence a person's consciousness. For example, a person can act out an unconscious fantasy that he or she is impervious to danger, a rough and tough risk-taker. A patient with this type of script may take chances unnecessarily and have a cavalier attitude about rehabilitation.

The retreat into a fantasy world is considered an immature defense mechanism and coping style, but for some patients with aphasia, it can be desirable, mature, and adaptive given the extreme circumstances (Tanner, 2010, 2012). For normal people, the autistic fantasy defense mechanism, when used in excess, can be socially undesirable, but for individuals with aphasia, it can bridge the gap between desire and unpleasant reality. It can help them obtain needed relief from social and communicative frustrations in their retreat into imaginary worlds.

Patients engaging in autistic fantasy escape may be misdiagnosed as distracted, blanking out, unresponsive, and unmotivated in rehabilitation. While it is true that some patients with neurogenic communication disorders may be unmotivated and have attentional disorders, especially those with traumatic brain injury, others may be escaping reality as an attempt to cope with psychological distress. Rather than being disengaged from a certain therapy because of neurological deficits, the patient may be withdrawing, fantasizing, and daydreaming as a symbolic way of meeting his or her psychological needs. The patient may be dealing with emotional conflicts, and experiencing a brief respite from the ego threats associated with confronting the disability in therapy. Of course, the use of fantasy escape by people with aphasia can also be maladaptive, socially undesirable, and interfere with optimal speech and language rehabilitation and other therapies. If the patient frequently avoids therapies and social interaction by engaging in fantasy escape, he or she will not benefit optimally from rehabilitation.

Normal people engage in autistic fantasy escapes using visual imagery facilitated by internal monologues. Simply put, people show themselves pictures and narrate stories using internal monologues. Global aphasia patients, because of language deprivation, are limited to visual imagery during fantasy escapes. However, the psychological defense mechanism and coping style of autistic fantasy can be successfully employed by language-deprived patients to satisfy their psychological needs.

Case Studies, Illustrations, and Examples: Autistic Fantasy

Another session of therapy. Sometimes, you feel that you are on a fast track to rehabilitation that gives you very little time to appreciate your successes. Today, your mission is to compute numbers correctly. You find the right number of quarters in a dollar, count ten pennies to make a dime, add one column of numbers, and subtract this, that, and the other thing. You are not doing well with these numbers. Once, they were so easily computed and now they seem monumental problems. A sense of failure overwhelms you. Whew! You stare at a door knob. For a few precious seconds, you see yourself in your back yard. Your Wheaton Terrier jumps to retrieve a well-thrown Frisbee. The freshly mown grass is green, flowers are blooming, and the white picket fence clearly marks the boundary of that wonderful place. You are once again normal. Again, you throw the Frisbee and the dog grasps it in its teeth. But the words, " ... would the loaf of bread cost?" bring you back to reality. As you, the dog, Frisbee, flowers, and grass dissolve in your mind, you now find yourself struggling to remember how many dimes in a dollar. At the end of the session, the clinician will write in the chart that you have difficulty attending to tasks. Table 3-1 shows avoidance and escape defense mechanisms and coping styles arising from predominantly external threats and stressors. Table 3-1 shows the avoidance and escape defense mechanisms and coping styles.

Table 3-1
Avoidance and Escape Defense Mechanisms and Coping Styles

PSYCHOLOGICAL DEFENSE AND COPING STYLE	DESCRIPTION	USE BY LANGUAGE-DEPRIVED PATIENT
Avoidance	Simple avoidance of perceived external threat	Yes
Ego Restriction	Abandonment of an activity in response to anxiety and threats to self-esteem	Yes
Physical Escape	Physical escape from a negative and threatening situation	Yes
Autistic Fantasy	Escape through daydreaming as a symbolic way of meeting psychological needs	Yes

Predominantly Internal Threats

There is no clear distinction between threats of an external and internal nature because perceived external dangers are also accompanied by the disturbing thoughts related to them. However, this distinction is important when discussing patients with aphasia because discovery and analysis of perceived threats and dangers are hindered because of the communication barrier. As noted above, when the perceived threats and dangers are primarily prompted by internal thoughts, feelings, drives, memories, and ideas, the defense mechanisms and coping styles involve denial, avoidance, or some other way of blocking, suppressing, or repressing them. The following defense mechanisms and coping styles are relevant to patients with neurogenic communication disorders, and most are at least partially available to language-impaired or global aphasic persons.

Denial

In Chapter 2, anosognosia was defined as the denial of disease or disability as a consequence of brain injury. However, denial is integral to many defense mechanisms and coping styles not resulting from brain damage. Denial can be organically based, as discussed previously, but also can occur as the initial stage in the grief response (see Chapter 4). Denial as a defense mechanism protects the ego, reduces anxiety, and keeps unacceptable thoughts, feelings, drives, memories, and ideas from conscious awareness.

Authorities on denial as a defense mechanism and coping style sometimes make a distinction between complete and partial denial. In partial denial, the person acknowledges some aspects of reality while minimizing them. However, partial denial is more likely the activation, at least partially, of rationalization, intellectualization, or other defense mechanisms and coping styles to deal with psychological distress. Denial protects the ego by blocking threatening and unpleasant events, memories, and situations from conscious awareness. Psychotic denial refers to a gross impairment in reality testing. It is considered a perceptual defense mechanism and coping style not requiring language (Tanner, 2003, 2010, 2012). As such, it is a natural and likely defense for language-deprived individuals.

There is sometimes a religious or spiritual theme to denial. Religion and spirituality can have a positive or a negative effect on a patient's mental health. Huttlinger and Tanner (1994) and Tanner and Huttlinger (1989) report the positive psychological effects of a Peyote Healing Ceremony on a traditional Navajo person with aphasia. Patients with an external frame of reference, those who believe many of life's experiences are caused or influenced by external forces, are often passive in their denial. They deny partially or completely their disability and attribute dysfunction to external forces. These individuals often discount the need to participate in medical treatment because they believe God, or another force, will make them whole again. They deny the reality of the situation and the realities associated with recovery.

Denial can be an effective tool to delay confrontation with psychological threats for patients without language. However, persistent use of denial is a negative prognostic factor for optimal speech and language rehabilitation. Patients who persistently engage in denial are unrealistic and may never fully confront their disabilities negating the benefits of rehabilitation. Denial is a radical defense requiring substantial psychological energy. It takes a great deal of psychological energy to deny some aspect of reality in the presence of clear evidence of its existence.

Patients in denial may also negatively affect the rehabilitation programs. If the patient does not believe he or she has a communication disorder, or other disability related to the neurological event, some rehabilitation team members may feel useless and ineffective in performing their duties. Their professional roles are threatened when a patient clearly in need of rehabilitation denies his or her disability and refuses treatment. Unfortunately, some rehabilitation professionals brutally confront the denying patient with the reality of his or her situation. In most cases this is counterproductive, and often causes the patient to be more fixated and rigid in his or her denial.

Case Studies, Illustrations, and Examples: Denial

The private practice company provided speech and hearing services to the regional hospital seven days a week, and completed dysphagia evaluations within 24 hours of referral. To provide weekend services to the rehabilitation center, the company utilized graduate students willing to work on weekends under the 100% supervision of a clinical supervisor. One Saturday, the supervisor and student clinician attempted to treat a patient who actively denied his communication disorders and the need for rehabilitation.

Earnest, a 66-year-old male, suffered a stroke resulting in severe dysarthria and mild aphasia, primarily word-finding difficulties. The unilateral upper motor neuron damage resulted in spastic dysarthria and rendered him only about 40% intelligible. The dysnomia was resolving rapidly and largely spontaneously. The patient also had hemiparesis on the right side of his body, and was on a choking and aspiration precaution program.

When the student clinician and supervisor entered the patient's room, they were greeted by him in a friendly and pleasant manner. When the student clinician prepared the flash cards for the rapid recall exercises and dysarthria drills, Earnest in a matter-of-fact manner, questioned the need for the therapy. Through distorted and barely intelligible speech, he communicated that there was: "Nothing wrong with him and that he was in the hospital only for routine tests." All efforts to convince him of his impairments were unsuccessful including replaying audio recordings of his dysarthric speech. He simply would not acknowledge his speech and language disorders. Only after the supervisor informed Earnest that if he did not participate in therapy, the student would receive an incomplete grade did he agree to take part in the therapeutic activities. Though initially he believed the activities were useless, toward the end of the session, he began to acknowledge several distorted speech sounds, reduced intelligibility, and wordfinding deficits.

Repression

Repression, an extremely important defense mechanism and coping style, is used to keep threatening or painful thoughts and desires from consciousness. Repression, like denial, is one of the more common defense mechanisms and coping styles, and is sometimes referred to as "motivated forgetting." Many defense mechanisms and coping styles are different manifestations of repression. Carlat (1999) described repression as "stuffing" the emotion out of conscious awareness.

Repression differs from suppression in that the former is done automatically and involuntarily. In repression, negative thoughts, feelings, drives, memories, and ideas are excluded from consciousness by inhibiting them before or after they reach a conscious level. In repression, they are attended to and stored, but recall is inhibited. Thus, negative thoughts, feelings, drives, memories, and ideas are inaccessible preventing unbearable anxiety. Some authorities believe "slips of the tongue" are the surfacing of subconscious repressed memories.

Repression may be one factor in the amnesia surrounding the cerebral insult experienced by many patients with neurogenic communication disorders. Many patients cannot remember the events immediately cooccurring with the stroke or traumatic brain injury. For example, they do not remember the car accident or collapsing to the floor from a stroke. While brain damage, particularly to the hippocampus, may be the physical basis for the post-traumatic or post-stroke selective amnesia, repression of the events surrounding the catastrophe can also contribute or account for the memory loss. The events are so psychologically traumatic, the patient represses them thus protecting himself or herself from unbearable anxiety.

Amnesia is associated with disruptions of neurochemicals. However, the memory deficits patients frequently experience regarding events surrounding the cerebral insult may also be related to repression of psychologically painful experiences. The patient may see illness as pure negativity and hardship. He or she may unconsciously interpret illness as a punishment for past sins or there may be a vague feeling of guilt.

> Often, however, the guilt-ridden patient who sees his illness as punishment fears that the fates have even more suffering in store for him. Such a person may have a prior history of constantly fearing that something bad is going to happen to him and reacts to physical illness as if the long-dreaded doomsday has arrived. (Imboden and Urbaitis, 1978, p. 30)

Therefore, the patient prone to repression has the tendency to expel and withhold from conscious awareness events surrounding the catastrophic event.

Brain damage may also undo repression and cause the patient to experience anxiety because previously repressed memories surface. For example, a patient with a traumatic brain injury may experience anxiety because he or she is unable to keep repressed painful thoughts about childhood from his or her conscious awareness. This return of the repressed can account for some anxious behaviors seen in patients with severe traumatic brain injuries and strokes and is called "the return of the repressed."

Psychotherapy, the "talking cure," addresses the failure of repression to prevent conscious awareness of negative thoughts, feelings, drives, memories, and ideas. Using the person's intact reasoning abilities and unimpaired memory, psychotherapists help analyze the repressed. The goal is to have the conscious ego examine the repressed information logically and maturely. Unfortunately, most patients with aphasia cannot benefit from psychotherapy due to the communication disorder and a loss of abstract attitude. An abstract attitude is necessary to reason and critically analyze issues related to repression. Patients with traumatic brain injuries may also lack the mental executive functioning necessary to benefit from psychotherapy. Repression is well within the range of language impaired or global aphasic persons, but psychotherapy is contraindicated for many patients with neurogenic communication disorders.

Case Studies, Illustrations, and Examples: Repression

The tragic car pileup occurred within the Flagstaff city limits one January afternoon. Mrs. Wannamaker and her husband were traveling from California to their new lives in Iowa. Only married for a few days, the young couple had left their jobs and were beginning anew. It was the second marriage for the couple and the two children from their previous marriages were secured safely in the backseat of the compact car. The blizzard had raged all day and visibility was less than twenty feet because of the heavy, wet snow. Creeping along at 20 miles per hour, the tractor-trailer truck in front of them jack-knifed causing their car to slide into its back wheels. Then, a dozen huge trucks and many cars crashed into each other. That cold wintery day in Flagstaff, Arizona, seven people lost their lives and Mrs. Wannamaker suffered a major closed head injury.

Nearly a year after the accident, Mrs. Wannamaker sued several trucking companies and their insurance companies for the injuries she suffered. During the depositions, it was discovered she had no memory of the accident. In fact, Mrs. Wannamaker could not remember the previous ten years of her life, her son, or that she was on her way to a new life in Iowa. She had only a vague sense of recognition of her new husband. During the depositions, experts testified that while much of her memory loss for the accident and the previous ten years of her life were caused by specific damage to parts of her brain, she had also likely repressed the memory of the tragic events that cost her so much. An expert witness in neuropsychiatry opined that the car pileup, deaths, and injuries were so violent and disturbing, the psychological repression of those events combined with the brain injury to cause the nearly complete ten-year retrograde amnesia. The case never went to court and the trucking and insurance companies compensated her for pain, suffering, and the loss of her memory.

Psychological Regression

Regression is a withdrawal to a more secure and comfortable level of adjustment. The patient engaged in regression as a defense mechanism and coping style returns to a manner of reaction to life's stressors that she or he has outgrown. It is usually a subconscious return to an immature stage of psychological adjustment to avoid anxiety and involves thoughts, behaviors, and emotions. Chapman (1976, p. 63) provided an example of total regression occurring in a woman who finds problems of marriage and child rearing overwhelmingly stressful: "She may flee into psychogenic physical symptoms that allow her to become a dependent, childlike invalid, and she thus frees herself from the complex responsibilities of marriage and child rearing which she finds overwhelming." In partial regression, a person may have some adult thoughts, behavior, and emotions, but retreats into childlike regression in specific situations.

As discussed previously, Joseph Wepman suggested that aphasia is a psycholinguistic regression affecting the patient's entire personality. For example, the speechlessness of an infant corresponds to global aphasia, semantic aphasia corresponds to the stage of vocabulary learning of a child, syntactic aphasia correlates with the grammatical acquisition stages in children, and so forth. According to Wepman, the recovery from aphasia should parallel the stages of language acquisition.

While Wepman's "linguistic regression theory" of aphasia has been discounted, some patients with aphasia do regress psychologically. They seek dependent relationships and find comfort in the immature role of a child, thus satisfying the need for security. In this discussion, the psychological defense and coping style of regression does not refer to the Freudian concepts of psychosexual development and fixations. As used here, regression is the return to earlier patterns of thoughts and behaviors that serve to protect the ego. As such, regression can be benign, and in the case of global aphasia, an understandable method of coping with adversity and protection of the ego.

Regression to the immature role of a dependent child may be understandable, adaptive, and appropriate, particularly during early stages of recovery, especially for severely involved patients. Importantly, regression does not require language to be utilized and is well within the range of aphasic patients, including globally involved persons. However, the goal of rehabilitation is to produce an independent and productive individual within the constraints of the communication disorder, so regression to dependency should be gradually discouraged.

Case Studies, Illustrations, and Examples: Psychological Regression

The weekly rehabilitation meetings begin at 7:00 AM every Thursday and are regularly attended by a physiatrist, medical social worker, speech-language pathologist, neuropsychologist, dietician, physical and occupational therapists, and several rehabilitation nurses. At the meetings, each rehabilitation patient's diagnosis, treatment plan, and progress are discussed in detail, and the weekly plans of treatment are established, reviewed, and adjusted where appropriate. The physiatrist begins the meeting with Ruby, a 56-year-old right-handed female, who suffered a dense occlusive stroke involving the frontal lobe of her left hemisphere. She presents with right hemiparesis, dysarthria, predominantly expressive aphasia, and moderately severe apraxia of speech. After providing the medical history, the physiatrist asks each member of the rehabilitation team to discuss the patient's progress during the past week.

The neuropsychologist reports that Ruby is depressed and anxious, and her physician has her on an antidepressant that also reduces anxiety. Her primary nurse indicates she refuses to dress or feed herself when her husband is present. She sometimes refuses to get out of bed unless her husband encourages her to do so. The occupational therapist notes that during meal times, she attempts to feed herself and is largely successful. Unfortunately, when her husband is present, she stops all attempts at independent eating, and requires he bring the food and liquid to her mouth while encouraging her to eat. The physical therapist observes that during transfers, Ruby attempts the exercises and improves unless her husband is present. When he is in the therapy gym, she sits limply in the wheelchair will not participate in the therapy unless assisted and encouraged by him. Concluding the status report for the patient, the speech-language pathologist notes that during therapies, Ruby attempts production of the sounds and recall of words, but when her husband is present, she is passive and looks to him to do the communicating.

The team agrees the patient regresses to a childlike and dependent state when her husband is present. The social worker indicates she will discuss the issue with Ruby's husband and counsel him in strategies to reduce her dependency on him. The rehabilitation team agrees to provide therapies in her husband's absence, and try to gradually reduce Ruby's dependency on him.

Passive-Aggression

A person engaged in the passive-aggressive defense mechanism and coping style appears timid, cautious, and shy, but indirectly expresses his or her anger, hostility, and aggression toward others, particularly authority figures. The passive-aggressive person wants approval and acceptance, but is offish, diffident, and aloof to mask the underlying hostility. A passive-aggressive person is angry, hostile, and aggressive, but these emotions and behaviors are presented in a passive and indirect way. Procrastination, lying, making excuses, sarcasm, and complaining are often signs of the passive-aggressive defense mechanism and coping style.

Patients with aphasia may engage in passive-aggression to cope with the lack of control over their disorder. For example, a patient with underlying anger, hostility, and aggression may appear to want to fully participate in rehabilitation, and agrees to complete therapeutic tasks. However, they will not follow through with them. Using the passive-aggressive defense mechanism and coping style, the patient copes with the demands and negativity of the communication disorder through passive, yet aggressive means. The behavior is seen in dealings with rehabilitation authority figures such as doctors, nurses, therapists, and others with whom the patient does not feel comfortable in confronting openly.

The chronic passive-aggressive patient often has trust issues and may fear intimacy which is often founded in early learning. Many rehabilitation therapies involve close physical contact and the analysis of previously private thoughts, attitudes, and behaviors. As such, a patient may passively resist these activities to prevent perceived intrusion into personal, intimate, and private aspects of his or her life. It is a passive, yet aggressive way of coping with negative and disturbing thoughts and feelings.

The passive-aggressive defense mechanism and coping style does not require language; it is largely a subconscious process. Passive-aggression is a "nonverbal" defense mechanism and coping style, thus, language-deprived, global aphasic patients can employ it. Passive-aggression may be apparent and obvious with the patient's actively resisting rehabilitation or more subtle where he or she feigns confusion and is obstructionistic regarding treatment programs and activities.

Case Studies, Illustrations, and Examples: Passive-Aggression

After several weeks of outpatient aphasia therapy, the clinician concluded the patient and his wife were angry, hostile, and engaged in aggressiveness through passive means. While occasionally being late for outpatient sessions is understandable, the patient and his wife consistently were twenty minutes late and several times, they did not show up nor did they call to cancel. At first, the clinician assumed the tardiness and absences were attributable to carelessness and difficulties getting to and from the hospital. However, both are physically independent and capable of making other appointments and recreational activities on time, often showing up beforehand.

The clinician understands that being a patient in a large medical facility is often frustrating what with schedules, parking, traffic, and all of the paperwork associated with receiving the services. A certain amount of complaining is understandable and even expected. Even in the best of facilities, patients are often treated as one small cog in a huge medical machine. Nevertheless, the complaints all seem to focus on the outpatient aphasia therapy. Over the past several weeks, the clinician sensed hostility from both the patient and his wife.

Part of the outpatient aphasia therapy involved extensive home assignments for word recall, writing, and simple arithmetic. At the end of each session, the clinician gave the patient and his wife detailed assignments and instructions on completing them. However, they rarely completed the home assignments always providing excuses and complaints that the instructions were vague and incomplete. Never did the patient or his wife openly show anger or hostility to the clinician; it was always subtle and covert.

Seeing the outpatient aphasia therapy was not effective, possibly because of unresolved anger and hostility, albeit indirectly and passively expressed, the clinician transferred the patient to another therapist hoping she would have better results. Several weeks later, the new speech-language pathologist reported better outcomes and responsiveness to the therapy.

Reaction Formation

Reaction formation is the substitution of attitudes and behaviors diametrically opposed to what the person feels and would like to do. Reaction formation is often seen as excessive behavior, e.g., being too friendly, ordered, cheerful, or generous. "Too much, too often" may signal that a person is engaging in reaction formation in an attempt to permanently relieve anxiety.

Reaction formation may drive a person to be a pornography fighter. The individual may become obsessed with eliminating pornography because it arouses him or her, and anxiety is reduced or eliminated by speaking and writing against it. Although an overused and overgeneralized label, "homophobic" attitudes and behaviors may hide deep-rooted feelings of homosexuality.

Sigmund Freud considered the trait of cleanliness one manifestation of a reaction formation. In excess, it may be a defense mechanism and coping style against the repressed desire to be cluttered and messy. Generosity can be a defense against unconscious stinginess, cheerfulness a reaction formation against underlying depression, and engaging in "daredevil" behavior may indicate deep-rooted repressed fears. The quote from Shakespeare's "Hamlet" succinctly captures the attitudes and behaviors of a person utilizing the reaction formation defense mechanism and coping style: "The lady doth protest too much, methinks."

Reaction formation is a difficult defense mechanism and coping style to understand because it appears counterintuitive. A good example of reaction formation is Stockholm syndrome where a hostage displays love, affection, and commitment to his or her abuser. In some instances, the person with the syndrome may willingly engage in criminal acts such as bank robbery. While Stockholm syndrome may involve several defense mechanisms and coping styles, it can also partially be explained by a reaction formation. It is an attempt by the hostage to cope with the complete control the terrorist or hostage-taker has over him or her. By embracing the terrorist or hostage-taker, anxiety and fear is reduced or eliminated.

All patients with neurogenic communication disorders can use reaction formation including language-deprived people. For example, a patient who is obsessively orderly may be using reaction formation to deal with deep-seated anxiety associated with the disorder and disorganization caused by the disability. Language, which brings order to thought, is lost in global aphasia, and some patients are excessively disturbed by untidy and unkempt hospital rooms and therapy suites. Such behavior can signal attempts by the patient to obtain relief from anxiety associated with the communication disorder. Certainly, not all excessive attitudes and behaviors are reaction formations, but in some patients with aphasia, they can suggest utilization of this defense mechanism and coping style.

Case Studies, Illustrations, and Examples: Reaction Formation

The clinician finds the patient to be pleasant, cooperative, and motivated during the aphasia therapy sessions. She is a good-natured woman with severe expressive and receptive language impairments cutting across all modalities of communication. However, at the conclusion of each session, the patient breaks from her typical pleasant and cooperative manner and becomes discomposed and agitated. Each time as the clinician prepares to leave the room, the patient makes noises and gestures indicating dissatisfaction and distress.

Initially, the clinician was baffled at the patient's change in affect after the sessions; she could not understand what prompted it. Was the patient offended by something the clinician had done during the session? Was she upset because the session was over? Was her anger directed at the clinician or the situation? For several weeks, the clinician could not understand the strange transition from the patient being cooperative and pleasant to being angry, demanding, and agitated. The clinician always tried to end aphasia therapy sessions on a positive note, and this was impossible with this particular patient. One day, almost by accident, the clinician discovered the source of the dramatic change in affect on the patient.

At the end of the session, and in an attempt to calm and comfort the patient, the clinician returned to her beside and patted her on the arm. Then, as the clinician was leaving, she returned the table used in therapy to its original position in the room and readjusted the water container, cup, and tray. The patient immediately calmed down and returned to her good-tempered self. Sensing the patient's agitation and anger resulted from her leaving the room in perceived disarray, at the end of the next therapy session, she carefully returned objects exactly to their original positions. This solved the problem and in future sessions, she was able to end them on a positive note. The clinician recognized that for the aphasic patient, the language disorder was anxiety-provoking and distressing because of the loss of order and predictability. By the clinician returning her room to its original, tidy state, the patient attained as much order and predictability as possible given the situation.

Displacement and Projection

Displacement and projection are combined in this discussion of defense mechanisms and coping styles because both involve redirecting or shifting anxiety-provoking thoughts, feelings, drives, memories, or ideas. Displacement is a subconscious attempt to reduce anxiety by shifting negative emotions from one person or object to another. As used here and in other discussions of defense mechanisms and coping styles, the subconscious is broadly defined and considered accessible to the conscious mind. In displacement, negative emotions are displaced to a neutral or less threatening or dangerous person or object. Hostile feelings for a supervisor at work can be displaced to a subordinate, and practical jokes can disguise feelings of hostility. Sometimes, patients and their families direct displacement toward therapists and nurses because doctors are too threatening to confront openly. They may take out their anger on other health care professionals when the source of it is a doctor. Throwing a water glass against a wall is an example of displacement of anger to an inanimate object. Typically, anger is displaced, but other emotions may also be redirected to a less threatening person or object.

Projection is a subconscious rejection of emotionally unacceptable thoughts, feelings, drives, memories, or ideas and the act of attributing them to someone else. In the extreme, delusions and hallucinations are psychotic projections of inner turmoil to the outside world. A projecting person subconsciously attributes his or her unacceptable thoughts, feelings, drives, memories, and ideas onto someone else. Projection reduces anxiety and guilt by blaming others for negative thoughts and emotions. An example of a projection defense mechanism and coping style is a person who believes his or her spouse is being unfaithful without evidence to support it. He or she may be projecting the desire for an extramarital relationship, which is emotionally unacceptable, onto his or her spouse.

Through projection, the patient's family members may sometimes allay anxiety and guilt they may have about their inability or unwillingness to care properly for their loved one. They may project that the members of the rehabilitation team do not provide proper therapies for their loved one, when in reality, the care is appropriate. Statements made by family members, such as "You don't seem to care whether he gets better or not," "You don't spend enough time with my mother," and "You don't put in as much time with my brother as you do with the other patients" may be projections of their own inadequacies and indifference. The patient may also indicate that a therapist does not seem motivated to provide quality therapy, when in fact, it is his or her lack of motivation being projected to the therapist. Of course, these statements and indications by family members and patients could be accurate appraisals of the situation.

Displacement and projection are capable of being used by language-deprived individuals. Language is not necessary to displace hostility and anger onto a safe person or object. Neither is language necessary to project one's own wishes, motivations, and emotions onto someone else. Both defense mechanisms and coping styles allow the person to avoid awareness of negative thoughts and emotions and to reduce anxiety.

Case Studies, Illustrations, and Examples: Displacement and Projection

The complaint against the rehabilitation team was brought to the hospital administration by the patient's son. He alleged that several doctors, nurses, and therapists abused his father by unnecessarily causing him pain, regularly ignoring his requests for pain medication, and neglecting to provide him with adequate rehabilitation services. The hospital administration took the complaint seriously and referred the case to the medical's staffs' professional conduct committee.

Each doctor, nurse, and therapist listed in the complaint met with the committee and responded to the allegations. All of the accused health care professionals denied them. The physical therapist agreed some of therapies to treat the patient's arm and leg paralysis may cause discomfort, but they were necessary, unavoidable, and consistent with the standards of practice. The patient's primary care physician noted that pain medications were available to the patient, adequate in the dosage, and within established prescription guidelines. Several nurses reported that never was the patient denied pain medication when he indicated the need for it. The speech-language pathologist and occupational therapist were perplexed at the complaints, and indicated there was no foundation to them. Fortunately, there were video recordings available which supported the rehabilitation team's defense. Other family members also questioned the allegations brought by their brother and told the committee they had no evidence that their father's treatment was substandard, abusive, or inadequate. In fact, they indicated the services were of high quality and having positive results. The committee noted that the son had only visited his father twice since his admission to the facility.

During the investigation, it was found that prior to the patient's admission to the rehabilitation facility, the son had been investigated for neglecting and abusing his invalid father, and was found to have been stealing his pain medication. There were also reports that he would physically punish his father for episodes of incontinence. After the thorough investigation, the professional conduct committee concluded the allegations were without merit and cleared the rehabilitation team of wrongdoing. The son was subsequently investigated for abuse and neglect of an incapacitated adult, and appropriate actions were taken by the social services department.

Altruism, Sublimation, and Substitution

Altruism, sublimation, and substitution are categorized together because they involve a person redirecting the negative to personally or socially acceptable thoughts, attitudes, and behaviors. They are similar defense mechanisms and coping styles used by persons to reduce anxiety. Persons using the altruism defense mechanism and coping style are self-sacrificing and receive satisfaction, gratification, and rewards from the responses of others. Sublimation is the acceptance of a socially approved substitute goal for a drive whose normal mode of expression is blocked. A person sublimating redirects an unwanted impulse into thoughts and actions that are positive or less malignant. Substitution, a more direct and less subtle defense mechanism and coping style, is used to reduce anxiety by substituting an unobtainable emotion, object, or goal with one that is more attainable and acceptable. It also involves disguising the motivations for doing something. When used appropriately, altruism, sublimation, and substitution are mature ways of dealing with negativity and can be used, more or less, by all people with aphasia.

The defense mechanism and coping style of altruism can be a mature, adaptive, and partially within the range of most patients with aphasia depending on the severity of the communication disorder and other disabilities. The mature and adaptive defense mechanism and coping style of altruism is different from "autistic surrender," a concept advanced by Anna Freud, where a person avoids anxiety by living vicariously and abandoning his own ambitions. An example of altruism is the patient who writes about his rehabilitation challenges, successes, trials, and tribulations. While authors write for many reasons, books about recovery of illness may be written for altruistic reasons. By helping others through writing, a person deals with the negative aspects of the communication disorder.

Sublimation is a mature, adaptive defense mechanism and coping style where unacceptable impulses or ideas are transformed into socially acceptable behaviors. Sublimation is the transfer or channeling of potentially harmful and negative psychological energy into personally or socially acceptable thoughts and actions. Engaging in sports allows people to sublimate aggressive and assertive urges. Sexual sublimation is seen in some religions where celibacy is required of the ministry. Celibacy permits the transformation of sexual impulses into good religious acts. An aphasic patient sublimating aggressive impulses may excel in physical therapy strengthening exercises as a way of venting anger and aggressive impulses. Therapists are familiar with the altruistic patient who is eager to help others and assumes the role of nurturer in group therapy sessions. Both sublimation and altruism involve the individual engaging in unselfish ways of channeling negativity.

Substitution closely resembles sublimation and altruism. Substitution is a response to frustration, and is employed to reduce anxiety and other negative emotions by disguising motivations. Substitution is a type of avoidance that permits an attainable or acceptable object, goal, or emotion for one that is blocked. Substitution, as used here, does not include the substitution of sexual desires to objects. A patient with facial paralysis may refuse to look in mirrors because of facial sag and drooling that leads to negative thoughts; thus, he or she substitutes younger pictures of himself or herself in lieu of mirrors. The substituting patient may feel deformed by a stroke, so he or she might put energy into being witty and humorous.

Sublimation, substitution and altruism are defenses capable of being employed by even patients suffering from severe neurogenic communication disorders. Even severely involved aphasic patients can sublimate, substitute, or be altruistic. Language is not required to engage in unselfish redirection of negative emotions and drives. These defenses can range from writing elaborately about the trials and tribulations of recovery to assisting others with speech drills within the confines of their own disabilities.

Case Studies, Illustrations, and Examples: Altruism, Sublimation, and Substitution

Prior to the stroke, Mr. Chuck Huston was a successful businessman and director of retail sales for a large company. He was an excellent public speaker and noted for his leadership abilities. At age 42, he suffered a stroke rendering him moderately aphasic and partially paralyzed on the right side of his body. For the remaining years of his life, he traveled the country and spoke to college students in communication sciences and disorders about stroke, aphasia, and their effects on survivors' quality-of-life.

At first, the professor of communication sciences and disorders was reluctant to have Mr. Huston speak to the graduate students. Citing time constraints and fear Mr. Huston's speech would not be substantive enough to warrant an entire hour for the guest lecture, the professor put off Mr. Huston's repeated requests to travel the hundreds of miles to speak to the students. But Mr. Huston was persuasive and for several years he spoke to students about the frustrations and challenges of being a stroke survivor with aphasia. Although Mr. Huston's speeches were often interrupted by bouts of emotional labile crying and with wordfinding problems, they were educational, powerful, and persuasive in advocating for the right of aphasic people.

Based on Mr. Huston's guest lectures and other experiences with people with aphasia, the professor drafted the Aphasic Patient's Bill of Rights (see Appendix A). It was presented as a poster to a convention of the American Speech-Language-Hearing Association (Tanner, 1986), included in a self-help book for stroke survivors and their families, and made available as a wall poster by a major publishing company. Mr. Huston was also a woodworker and made several wall clocks on polished driftwood with the Aphasic Patient's Bill of Rights laminated on them. For the remaining years of his life, Mr. Huston promoted the Aphasic Patient's Bill of Rights in speeches at aphasia support groups and as a guest lecturer in college courses on the communication disorder.

Dissociation

Dissociation is the separation of emotional significance from an idea or situation and compartmentalizing of a person's consciousness or identity to minimize anxiety. According to the American Psychiatric Association (2013), it is also the separation of an idea from its emotional significance and affect. Dissociation is the detachment of a group of behavioral or mental processes from the rest of the person's consciousness. In extreme cases, it can lead to multiple personalities. Although most people occasionally dissociate, such as intently daydreaming, when done frequently and in excess, it is a radical, desperate attempt to cope with stressors. Dissociation is a detachment from reality and not the break from it, as seen in psychotic episodes. Dissociation allows a person to remove painful emotions from conscious awareness rather than to feel the pain. There are six types of dissociation relevant to people with aphasia: amnesia, depersonalization, fainting, fugue state, somnambulism, and multiple personality.

As reported previously, organic or psychological factors may cause amnesia. The retrograde amnesia experienced by some patients can involve repression of traumatic events, and be a reason why many patients dissociate and cannot remember the trauma or medical emergency that caused their injury. When psychologically based, dissociative amnesia is a person's attempt to separate himself or herself from painful information or experience. The selective memory loss relieves anxiety and negative emotions associated with the information or experience. Dissociative amnesia allows the person to forget people and events and to structure a world not contaminated with negative memories.

Depersonalization can be acute or chronic. It is an altered perception of experience including the sensation that one's identity or some aspect of it is detached from the body. In depersonalization, the individual may feel he or she is an observer looking at the world from above or outside. It can include feeling that one is in a dream, temporal distortions, and physically numbing (American Psychiatric Association, 2013). Derealization is similar to depersonalization and involves a person perceiving the world as not being real. It can also include perceptions of individuals and objects as unreal, lifeless, dreamlike, foggy, or visually distorted (American Psychiatric Association, 2013). In aphasia, it is easy for the patient to feel detached and sensing that he or she is living in an unreal situation. Especially early post-onset, the patient finds himself or herself in unusual, uncommon, and extraordinary circumstances. Ambulance transports, intensive care units, hospital rooms, and high technology imaging procedures are environmental changes and situations that can predispose, precipitate, and perpetuate feelings of being removed, detached, and living in an unreal situation.

Fainting, or syncope, is the temporary loss of consciousness. Of course, fainting may be caused by many medical factors such as low blood pressure, stroke, and dehydration. Fainting can also be a psychological defense mechanism and coping style, and serve as a radical but successful way of dissociating from reality. While rare, it may occur in aphasic patients suffering extreme catastrophic reactions. As Eisenson (1984, pp. 187-188) observed, during a catastrophic reaction, a patient may faint: "Vascular changes, irritability, evasiveness, or aggressiveness may precede or accompany the catastrophic reaction. An extreme catastrophic reaction may take the form of loss of consciousness." Psychologically, it is the complete shutdown of the ego and the attempt by the patient to separate himself or herself from the environment.

Dissociative fugue, also known as a "fugue state" or "psychogenic fugue" may occur in people suffering from seizures, dementia, and the effects of hallucinogenic drugs. However, when psychologically-based, it is a massive dissociation of personality resulting in the need to seek physical escape. The person in a fugue state may lose identity, become disoriented, experience confusion, and have dissociative amnesia. Often, it is associated with wandering and spontaneous travel. Usually, a person only has one episode of a psychogenic fugue state and most individuals have complete return to normalcy. Fugue states can last for hours, weeks, months, and even years. While rare, dissociative fugue states can occur in aphasic persons and are associated with seizures. However, because of the communication disorder, it is difficult to know when a patient is experiencing dissociative fugue and the extent of it.

Somnambulism is walking while asleep. It is common in children, but in adults, it may be an indication of psychological conflicts. It is associated with dreaming physically active fantasies. Some patients who fall out of bed at night may have done so because they were attempting to walk in their sleep. Most individuals who walk while asleep have little if any recollection of doing so. Somnambulism is associated with migraines, seizure disorders, schizophrenia, and anxiety disorders, and when psychologically based, it is considered a dissociative disorder. Somnambulism requires normal physical functions to perform and many patients with aphasia may be unable to engage it.

A person with multiple personalities, sometimes labeled "dissociative identity disorder," lives two or more lives independently without awareness of the others. The dissociation, a failure to integrate aspects of his or her personality, is thought to result from extreme and repeated childhood physical or sexual abuse. The true multiple personality disorder is rare, and some authorities question whether it exists as a clinical entity. Some psychiatrists and psychologists note that it is only discovered under hypnosis and may be an attempt on the part of the person to please the hypnotist or because of suggestion. Due to the communication barrier in aphasic patients, discovering whether a person is experiencing multiple personalities is difficult.

Case Studies, Illustrations, and Examples: Dissociation

Your eyes slowly open to unfamiliar sights, smells, and sounds. Even the crisp sheets covering you feel unusual. You survey the room and see it is some sort of futuristic bridge on a Starship. You see through the dimly-lit high-tech instruments beeping, flashing, buzzing, and humming to some undecipherable rhythm. All the instruments have one thing in common; they are connected by tubes, lines, and cords to your body. There is the irritation of the much-too-wide catheter tube.

There is an ever-present smell of disinfectant saturating the room. Outside, you hear matter-of-fact conversations punctuated by occasional laughter. You survey your body and feel the numbness. You will your right arm and leg to move, but motion is not forthcoming. Panic sets in as you struggle to break the confines of your left arm which is tightly restrained by white cloth strips secured to the bed's railing. You suspect you are in a hospital room, and shout to the powers-that-be "Help me." But adding insult to apparent injury, no words come to mind and no sounds leave your lips. You have a vague recollection of a fall to the floor and an ambulance ride. Finally, in retreat, you surrender and lie back on the stiff pillow. As a temporary reprieve from fear and confusion, you simply distance yourself from the here and now. It is all so unreal, and you bask in the relief that comes from dissociating yourself from this new terrible reality.

DEFENSE MECHANISMS AND COPING STYLES COMPROMISED IN APHASIA

As noted previously, the role language plays in the adjustment to aphasia has been theorized for decades. John Hughlings Jackson applied the concept of inner speech to the study of aphasia. He believed that all forms of speech were similar and that internal monologues occur with the same structure as other propositional utterances. Jackson believed it was artificial to consider the kind of utterance spoken to someone else as basically different from the utterances we speak to ourselves. Macdonald Critchley explored the use of inner symbols in aphasic patients and postulated the existence of a grammar to internal monologues (inner speech). He also postulated a "silent" nonverbal thinking process he called the "preverbitum" corresponding to visual and spatial problem-solving. Russell Brain concluded that aphasia must be considered on a psychological level.

People with aphasia have special adjustment challenges not experienced by those with intact language ability. Global aphasic people are unable to engage several defense mechanisms and coping styles that require the use of language. Even patients with partially intact language abilities are compromised and hindered in the use of verbal defense mechanisms and coping styles. Language is necessary, either externalized through discourse with others, or as a problem-solving function using internal monologues, when employing verbal defense mechanisms and coping styles. Rationalization, intellectualization, suppression, undoing, and humor are primarily verbal defense mechanisms and coping styles, and consequently are beyond the capabilities of most language-deprived individuals.

Rationalization and Intellectualization

Rationalization and intellectualization are often used synonymously as defense mechanisms and coping styles to elevate self-esteem by disguising motivations, making excuses, and masking feelings. Technically intellectualization is one form of rationalization, which is excessive reasoning to block disturbing emotions. It is seeking sanctuary in reason and isolating emotions from an act or behavior; emotionally removing the person from anxiety-provoking thoughts. It is sometimes called "flight into reason" and "isolation of affect."

Rationalization, in the broadest sense, is a conscious attempt by a person to make behaviors and emotions acceptable. It is often considered a face-saving device which relieves guilt and anxiety temporarily, and is sometimes considered as "making excuses." Whether dealing with acts of commission or omission, a person consciously justifies his or her action or inaction by attending to acceptable reasons for them and ignoring or denying unacceptable ones. When rationalization is truthful, and intellectualization is based on fact, these attempts by the ego to integrate and accept behaviors and emotions can be mature and adaptive. When used inappropriately, rationalization and intellectualization can restrict functioning and emotional adjustment.

Global aphasic patients, those individuals without language, are unable to use rationalization and intellectualization. Both defense mechanisms and coping styles are verbal and require language. Patients with global aphasia are unable to elevate self-esteem and relieve guilt and anxiety through rationalization and intellectualization. Patients with partial aphasia, depending on the degree of language deprivation, can employ rationalization and intellectualization in certain circumstances.

Case Studies, Illustrations, and Examples: Rationalization and Intellectualization

The aphasic patient was obviously having problems adjusting to the communication disorders. According to his wife, he was depressed, anxious, and had reduced self-esteem. She noted he felt worthless and useless especially during aphasia therapy when confronted with his impairments and limitations. Based on her report, the clinician decided to engage in externally imposed rationalizations to help the patient benefit from aphasia therapy.

During therapy, the clinician provided rationalization statements in situations where the patient displayed anxiety and low self-esteem due to poor speech and language performance. Statements made by the clinician such as, "I am sorry, I presented the material too rapidly," "My fault, you did fine," and "It is OK, there is too much distraction and noise in the room" appeared to help the patient rationalize his unsuccessful performance; thus, helping protect his ego and self-esteem. For externalized rationalizations to be effective, the patient's auditory comprehension was considered, and proper adjustments to the length and complexities were made to the statements. In addition, the externalized rationalizations were truthful, conducive to ego self-protection, and used sparingly.

Suppression

Suppression, a form of avoidance, is the voluntary exclusion of thoughts from conscious awareness. Repression differs from suppression in that the former is largely automatic and subconscious, while the latter is deliberate and conscious. In suppression, negative thoughts, feelings, drives, memories, or ideas are intentionally excluded from the person's consciousness. Suppression is making a conscious decision to avoid completely or delay attention to a thought, feeling, drive, memory, or idea in order to function in present reality.

Patients with aphasia may need to exclude from conscious awareness thoughts, feelings, drives, memories, or ideas related to the verbal impotence they experience because of wordfinding deficits, auditory comprehension impairments, dyslexia, unintelligible speech, and so forth. They may also need to suppress the thoughts associated with loss of the integrity of the self, rejection from others, the potential of further medical complications, and the possibility of death. Unfortunately for global aphasic patients, suppression primarily depends on exercising mental executive control over internal monologues. As a consequence, suppression for language-deprived patients may be ineffective or impossible. In addition, the perseverating patient (see chapter 2) may find suppression, as an adaptive, mature defense mechanism and coping style, compromised. However, early initiation of treatment may counter the negative effects of perseveration, and help the patient break from persistent negative and counterproductive thoughts.

Darley (1982, p. 177), in the first comprehensive review of the efficacy of aphasia therapy, reported: "Early initiation of treatment results in significantly greater improvement than results when treatment is delayed." While there are many reasons why patients with aphasia benefit more from early rather than delayed treatment, creating a positive mental set early post-onset may be a major one. Especially in patients with the tendency to perseverate, early initiation of treatment with the support, encouragement, and reinforcements associated with it, may counter the natural tendency to perseverate on the negative.

Case Studies, Illustrations, and Examples: Suppression

It seems everyone who enters the hospital room has a need to quiz you: "Do you know me?", "Is this a pen?", "Can you understand me?", "Do you know what this is?", "Do you know what happened to you?", "Do you know where you are?" It is not enough to always be barraged with these inane questions, it appears they must be shouted as if there is something wrong with your perfectly normal ears. Apparently, doctors, nurses, therapists, and even family members believe constantly quizzing you is the same as helping you.

Of course, you know where you are and what happened. And yes, you do have some trouble understanding the words of others, but that seems to be getting better every day. What is bothering you the most are the unrelenting words floating around in your head, and the gut-wenching feeling they cause. You just can't seem to stop them: "I'm brain damaged." You first overheard that pronouncement in the intensive care unit, and can't seem to stop it from circling around in your head. "I'm brain damaged" is a constant voice you can't seem to shake. It is like that tune you hear in the morning and can't stop the replay in your head. It seems the harder you try to shift that negative inner statement to something positive, the more resistant it is.

The speech-language pathologist understands your predicament and showers you with positive statements: "You're doing great," "You are getting better every day," "You're OK," "You are improving." Lately, you seem to have these positive thoughts taking the place of that damnable negative one. They seem to be antidotes to poisonous thoughts. It also appears that the positive inner statements also result in positive feelings: "I AM doing great," "I AM getting better every day," "I AM OK." Now, if people would just stop testing you.

Undoing

Undoing is an attempt through action or communication to take back an unacceptable behavior or thought. The action or communication is an attempt to partially or completely undo a previous one. Psychologically, the person attempts to deal with emotional conflicts by making amends. It is a symbolic defense mechanism and coping style. As used here, undoing is not limited to taking back an unconscious behavior or thought.

Since undoing is a ritualistic, symbolic act, it is likely unavailable to global aphasic patients. Global aphasic patients tend to be on a concrete level due to the loss of language. As reported previously, Kurt Goldstein is best known for postulating an abstract-concrete imbalance in aphasic patients' performance of reasoning tasks. Goldstein theorized that the aphasic patient has specific deficiencies in maintaining an abstract attitude. This loss of abstract attitude was present, not only in language, but in nonverbal performance tasks such as sorting colors and classifying objects. Goldstein viewed the aphasic patient as one suffering from a concrete attitude, bound to immediate experience, and lacking initiative and spontaneity.

Undoing also may be unavailable as a defense mechanism and coping style to language-deprived patients because it requires good communication skills and physical abilities to perform successfully. Therefore, undoing a previously unacceptable behavior may be impossible because the patient lacks the means to do it.

Case Studies, Illustrations, and Examples: Undoing

The patient was obviously distraught. She resisted transferring from her room to the dining room for therapy. You had intended to use food and utensils for stimuli and reinforcement for her wordfinding and grammatical problems. Ordinarily, the patient was cooperative, but yesterday's catastrophic reaction was unexpected and violent. It was so out-of-character for the patient. In retrospect, you should have noted the signs of her frustration and anxiety. About half way through the session, she pushed the tray on your lap and tried to hit you with her fist. Fortunately, you were able to avoid contact and several nurses and aides helped restore order. You dreaded today's session and a possible repeat of yesterday's disaster. As you approach the patient, she cheerfully attempts a greeting. She smiles and pats your hand in an obvious attempt to undo her negative actions of the previous day. Throughout the session, she cheerfully attends to each therapy exercise, always smiling, and doing her upmost even with the most challenging of requests.

Humor

The appreciation and use of humor as an overt expression of emotions is a mature psychological defense and coping style. In the humor defense mechanism and coping style, an amusing aspect of a stressor is emphasized. Prazich (1985, p. 29), a dentist who suffered a cerebral vascular accident with an accompanying neurogenic communication disorder, states:

> After a stroke, it is very hard not to be scared and feel sorry for yourself. A very good prescription for both of these feelings is laughter. As a result of losing control of my emotions, I discovered I felt really great inside after a good laugh. I knew this had some actual therapeutic value.

Of course, all displays of humor are not psychological defense mechanisms and coping styles, but humor can be used as a way of dealing with the pain of a neurogenic communication disorder.

Most types of humor, with the exception of slapstick and cartoons, require good language skills to use and appreciate. Many types of humor involve using language in unexpected ways. Consequently, language-deprived patients may be unable to use and appreciate humor when presented in lengthy jokes, monologues, and plays. Some humor requires abstraction and the concrete-abstract imbalance discussed previously may hinder the patient's use and appreciation of high-level witticisms. Humor as a psychological defense and coping style for many global aphasic patients is compromised due to impaired language comprehension and expression. For patients capable of employing humor as a defense mechanism and coping style, it may be effective for combating reduced self-esteem associated with aphasic errors the patient feels are embarrassing.

Case Studies, Illustrations, and Examples: Humor

A patient suffered a stroke about ten months ago, and had the typical wordfinding problems experienced by most patients with a predominantly expressive aphasia. Most errors had a "rhyme or reason" to them. The literal paraphasias, approximation errors, rhymed with the correct word. For example, when asked "What do you write with," he responded, "A hen." On another occasion, when asked the same question, he responded with the word "pencil," when in fact, he was pointing to a pen. The wordfinding error was a verbal paraphasia or an association error; it had a semantic association.

You and the patient share a love of deep sea fishing. You had gone sportfishing earlier in the week, and as promised, you brought him several cleaned and fileted yellowtail fish. He was obviously happy to receive the fish and remarked how tasty they would be. As you walked to the door of his house and bid him farewell, he said: "Thanks for the yellowtail, come back refrigerator and I'll cook them." He had erred by saying the apparently unrelated word, "refrigerator," for "tomorrow." The so-called "random" error came out of the blue and there was no apparent rhyme or reason to it. Then, almost automatically, he joked "Refrigerator–who said that?" The comment brought lighthearted laughter to both of you. Afterwards, you suspected the anomic error as not truly random; it was a result of him looking at his refrigerator when talking. The image of his refrigerator contaminated the word retrieval process. Regardless of the genesis of the paraphasia, the humor defused what would have been an awkward and embarrassing communication error. Table 3-2 shows psychological defenses and coping styles and the likelihood of them being compromised in language-deprived patients.

TABLE 3-2
PSYCHOLOGICAL DEFENSES AND COPING STYLES

PSYCHOLOGICAL DEFENSE AND COPING STYLE	DESCRIPTION	USE BY LANGUAGE-DEPRIVED PATIENTS
Denial	Blocking from conscious awareness of threatening and unpleasant events and situations	Yes
Repression	Excluding from conscious awareness negative thoughts, feelings, drives, memories, and ideas by inhibiting them before or after they reach a conscious level	Yes
Psychological Regression	Retreat to a more secure and comfortable level of adjustment	Yes
Passive-Aggression	Expressing anger, hostility, and aggression toward others in a passive way	Yes
Reaction Formation	Substitution of attitudes and behaviors that are diametrically opposed to actual ones	Yes
Displacement and Projection	Subconscious attempt to reduce anxiety by shifting negative emotions from one person or object to another or attributing them to someone else	Yes
Altruism, Sublimation, and Substitution	Redirecting the negative to personally or socially acceptable thought, attitudes, and behaviors	Yes
Dissociation	Detachment of a group of behavioral or mental processes from the rest of the person's consciousness	Yes, but difficult to determine in some patients with neurogenic communication disorders
Rationalization and Intellectualization	Attempts to elevate self-esteem and avoid disturbing emotions by disguising motivation and masking feelings	Compromised or unavailable
Suppression	Voluntary exclusion of thoughts from conscious awareness	Compromised especially in perseverative patients

(continued)

TABLE 3-2 (CONTINUED) PSYCHOLOGICAL DEFENSES AND COPING STYLES		
PSYCHOLOGICAL DEFENSE AND COPING STYLE	DESCRIPTION	USE BY LANGUAGE-DEPRIVED PATIENTS
Avoidance	Simple avoidance of perceived external threat	Yes
Undoing	An attempt through action or communication to take back an unacceptable behavior or thought	Compromised or unavailable
Humor	The appreciation and use of humor as an overt expression of emotions; emphasizing an amusing aspect of a conflict or stressor	Compromised or unavailable

CHAPTER SUMMARY

Defense mechanisms and coping styles are important in maintaining self-esteem and protection from disturbing thoughts, feelings, drives, memories, or ideas. Some are mature and adaptive while others are immature, maladaptive, neurotic, and radical attempts to cope with threats and stressors. Although the nature of coping styles and psychological defenses are the subject of continuing debate, the fact remains that people engage in them for psychological protection, and patients with aphasia are no exception. Global aphasic patients can use many defense mechanisms and coping styles, but some are compromised or unavailable because they require language. As stressors and threats to self-esteem increase, patients with aphasia may utilize more immature, maladaptive, neurotic, and radical attempts to adjust to them.

REFERENCES

American Psychiatric Association. (2013). *Diagnostic and statistical manual of mental disorders* (5th ed.). Arlington, VA: American Psychiatric Association.

Carlat, D. (1999). *The psychiatric interview*. Philadelphia, PA: Lippincott, Williams & Wilkins.

Chapman, A. (1976). *Textbook of clinical psychiatry*, (2nd ed.). Philadelphia, PA: Lippincott, Williams & Wilkins.

Darley, F. (1982). *Aphasia*. Philadelphia, PA: Saunders.

Eisenson, J. (1984). *Adult aphasia*, (2nd ed.). Englewood Cliffs, NJ: Prentice-Hall.

Halim, M., and Sabri, F. (2013). Relationship between defense mechanisms and coping styles among relapsing addicts. *The 3rd World Conference on Psychology, Counseling and Guidance*, 84, July 9, pp. 1829-1837.

Huttlinger, K., and Tanner, D. (1994). The peyote way: Implications for culture care theory. *Journal of Transcultural Nursing, 5*(2), 5-11.

Imboden, J., and Urbaitis, J. (1978). *Practical psychiatry in medicine*. New York, NY: Appleton-Century-Crofts.

Millon, T., and Meagher, S. (2004). The millon clinical multiaxial inventory-III (MCMI-III). In M. Hilsenroth, D. Segal (Eds.), *Comprehensive handbook of psychological assessment, Volume 2: Personality assessment*. Hoboken, NJ: John Wiley & Sons.

Porcerelli, J., and Hibbard, S. (2004). Projective assessment of defense mechanisms. In *Comprehensive handbook of psychological assessment, Volume 2: Personality assessment*. M. Hilsenroth and D. Segal (Eds). Hoboken, NJ: John Wiley & Sons.

Porcerelli, J., Thomas, S., Hibbard, S., and Cogan, R. (1998). Defense mechanisms development in children adolescents, and late adolescents. *Journal of Personality Assessment, 71*(3), 411-420.

Prazich, M. (1985). *A stroke patient's own story.* Danville, IL: Interstate Printers and Publishers.

Tanner, D. (1986). *The aphasic patient's bill of rights.* Paper presented at the Annual Convention of the American Speech and Hearing Association, Detroit, MI.

Tanner, D. (2003, Winter). Eclectic perspectives on the psychology of aphasia. *Journal of Allied Health,32*(4), 256-260.

Tanner, D. (2010). *Exploring the psychology, diagnosis, and treatment of neurogenic communication disorders.* New York, NY: iUniverse.

Tanner, D. (2012). Defense mechanisms and coping styles in aphasia. In R. Goldfarb (Ed.), *Translational speech-language pathology and audiology: Essays in honor of Dr. Sadanand Singh* (pp. 301-306). San Diego, CA: Plural

Tanner, D., and Huttlinger, K. (1989). *Peyote in the treatment of post traumatic aphasia: A case study.* Paper presented at the Annual Meeting of the American Society for Applied Anthropology. Santa Fe, NM.

Wallerstein, R. (1999). *Psychoanalysis: Clinical and theoretical.* Madison, CT: International Universities Press.

Appendix A

*Aphasic Patient's Bill of Rights**

Preamble

I am an individual with a speech and language disorder. The disorder may be mild and only cosmetically affect my ability to communicate or it may be severe and completely eliminate my ability to represent my thoughts and feelings with speech and language. My disorder can be complicated by sensory, perceptual, cognitive and psychiatric disturbances. I may be mobile, homebound or confined to a nursing home, medical care facility, hospital or rehabilitation center. Regardless of my deficits, I am entitled to the human dignity afforded to non-communicatively disabled individuals. Although my fundamental human rights are protected by the Constitution of the United States of America and other rights are extended to me by the policies and procedures of facilities and organizations, because of my communicative deficits, I require the following:

Our Relationship

Upon your acceptance of me as a patient, you assume three responsibilities. First, you are to provide the best clinical services of which you are capable. You are to use all of the knowledge, skills and resources available to help me minimize this disability. Second, by accepting me as your patient you agree to serve as my advocate in situations where I, my family or my court appointed guardian cannot represent my wishes. In those situations you will use your powers of speech and language to defend and protect me from attempts to deprive me of human dignity. Third, you have an obligation to provide significant people who come into contact with me your appraisal of my specific impairments and strengths. You will provide me with the benefit of the doubt regarding the status of those abilities which you are not absolutely certain have been impaired. Although I value and respect your professional position, you are employed by me. As such, my wishes will prevail regarding the course of therapy and all other considerations affecting me. If I am considered legally incompetent, my guardian will serve as my advocate, but this Bill of Rights will stand as a guiding principle for your interaction with me.

Unconditional Positive Regard

You have the responsibility to treat me with unconditional positive regard. You may not like or approve the things I say or do, but you have the responsibility to value me as a human being. You will project unconditional positive regard to me verbally, nonverbally and in all aspects of our relationship. In addition, because I may not be able to protest forced interaction with people who do not maintain positive regard for me, you will serve as my advocate in those situations. You will insure that I am protected and insulated from individuals who do not extend to me this basic human consideration.

Common Courtesy

I have the right to all of the common courtesies extended to the verbal population. I have the right to be addressed formally as Mr., Mrs., Ms., or Miss. I expect to be greeted in a pleasant and respectful manner. You shall engage in the social graces with me. I may not comprehend the words you speak, but I can appreciate the extension of common courtesy.

Grooming

I have the right to proper grooming. I shall be given adequate time to prepare myself for public interaction. If I am incapable of grooming myself due to paralysis or other impairments, I shall be assisted in becoming presentable. You have the responsibility not to transport me out of my room or home without addressing my right to proper appearance. Additionally, you will serve as my advocate to ensure that I will be presentable at all times.

Privacy

I have the right to privacy. I am entitled to periods alone or with relatives and friends. I have the right to have these times uninterrupted. I also have the right to refuse visitors. You have the responsibility to attend to my wishes regarding these matters and to protect my privacy.

Mobility

Although I may be confined to a wheelchair, I have the right to determine my movement. I have the right to be asked or encouraged to participate in decisions regarding mobility. You will not allow me to be "shuffled" from place to place without first informing me of the destination and, in some manner, obtaining my approval.

Emotions

I have the right to genuine, albeit in some cases, exaggerated emotions regarding my predicament without having them ignored or intellectualized as inappropriate. My emotions about this disability are appropriate to me and others should appreciate and respond appropriately to them. You have the responsibility to accept my emotions as genuine and to respond to them in an understanding and compassionate manner.

Personality

I have the right to my unique personality. As long as my behaviors are not destructive, I have the right to tolerance, understanding and appreciation of my unique personality characteristics. You have the responsibility to ensure that I am provided the same degree of personality tolerance extended to members of the verbal population.

Therapy

I have the right to be treated as an adult. Therapy materials designed for children are demeaning to me. You have the responsibility to insure that therapy materials are appropriate for my age, sex, interest, and disabilities.

I have the right to be informed of the prognosis for my recovery as a result of the therapy you provide to me. If I am incapable of understanding these reports, you have the responsibility to share the prognosis with my physician, family, or court appointed guardian.

I have the right to refuse therapy. A verbal person's wishes regarding therapy would be honored and I have the same rights.

I have the right to be made aware of the purposes of therapy techniques in those conditions where I am capable of comprehending all or part of them. We are partners in my treatment and you should attempt to communicate to me the objectives of a particular therapy. If behavior modification is used, I shall be made aware of the nature and purpose of the system. Foods, institutional privileges and other reinforcements may be used only with my (or my family's or guardian's) prior consent.

Quality Institutional Services

I have the right to prompt and considerate institutional services. Because "the squeaky wheel gets the grease," I may be denied the quality services provided to individuals with intact powers of speech and language. You will serve as my advocate to insure that I am treated fairly and provided quality services while I am disabled.

Dedicated to the memory of Mr. "Chuck" Huston.

Psychology of Aphasia

The Grief Response

"When you are sorrowful look again in your heart, and you shall see in truth you are weeping for that which has been your delight."

Kihlil Gibran

CHAPTER PREVIEW

This chapter examines the grief response in patients with aphasia. Loss of person, self, and object are discussed relative to patients with this neurogenic communication disorder. Loss of productive use of time, innocence, and gradual developmental loss are also reviewed. In this chapter, there is an examination of the stages many patients with aphasia pass through including a discussion of controversial aspects of the stage model of grieving. Grieving denial, responses to frustration (anger and bargaining), grieving depression, and acceptance are reviewed including suggestions to facilitate the patient's resolution of losses, and actions that can interrupt the process of reaching acceptance of them.

APHASIA AND UNWANTED CHANGE

On the most basic level, acquiring aphasia is being subjected to unwanted change. This unwanted change involves loss of valued persons, objects, and aspects of self. Although the patient may not physically lose loved ones because of the neurogenic communication disorder, such as occurs through death, divorce, departure, or separation, impaired or lost speech and language abilities frequently result in social detachment from loved ones. Loss of some aspect of self involves the inability or impaired ability to communicate, and the physical disabilities often cooccurring with aphasia such as walking and swallowing. As a result of the communication disorder and physical

Tanner, D.C.
The Psychology of Aphasia: A Practical Guide for Health Care Professionals
(pp 81-102). © 2017 Taylor & Francis Group.

disabilities, patients can be separated from valued objects such as home, car, pet, garden, library, recreation vehicles, and other objects with real and symbolic value.

Not all aphasias are of the severity to result in significant disabilities for the patient, but many do result in grievous losses, and the human reaction to unwanted change–the grief response (Tanner, 1980, 2003, 2006, 2008, 2009; Tanner, 2003; Tanner and Gerstenberger, 1996). Spillers (2007) and Code, Hemsley, and Herrmann (1999) report the grief model is important to understanding the emotional and psychosocial issues in patients with communication disorders.

Change involving loss begins early and occurs throughout a person's life. The infant loses comfort and security during feedings when he or she is weaned. The birth of another sibling can cause a sense of loss for the only-child. Young adults lose independence and freedom as family and society require more responsibilities. Divorce and separation are frequent occurrences in modern society. People lose valued assets because of untimely investments. Homes and possessions can be lost to fire, theft, and floods. As people age, developmental loss occurs as they lose hearing, sight, perceived attractiveness, physical mobility, and sexual desire and function. Humans are mortal, destined to die, and ultimately lose all worldly connections and life itself. According to the American Psychiatric Association (2013), bereavement refers to a range of grief and mourning responses associated with loss through death.

Both young and old people experience gradual developmental loss. Generally, for infants and children, the losses are not as painful because they are easily and rapidly replaced by other aspects of life. Major loss during childhood is also a predisposing factor for adult depression. Older people become more aware of the aging process, and the resulting developmental losses that accompany it.

Typically, developmental loss is gradual, but it can be brought rapidly into the consciousness of the patient with aphasia by the onset of the communication disorder. The patient may feel suddenly that he or she is aging too fast and irrevocably. He or she can be expected to grieve over this process, natural though it is. Nevertheless, loss is a natural consequence of living, and so is the grief response. For many patients with aphasia, unwanted change is around every corner:

> Loss of self occurs because of loss of the abilities such as walking, talking, dressing, and bowel and bladder control. Loss of person is the psychological separation the patient experiences from family and friends due to the communication disorder, and also because of physical placement in a nursing home or other type of extended care facility. Loss of object includes the use of a motor home, car, sewing machine, computer, or other valued object or pet due to physical and cognitive limitations and/or placement in a nursing home. (Tanner, 2007, p. 80)

Adjustment to aphasia shares similarities to coping with other chronic medical conditions. It is important to emphasize that the sense of loss experienced by patients with aphasia is dependent on their awareness levels. For example, patients with traumatic brain injury or stroke who have reduced or impaired awareness are unlikely to perceive the loss of person, objects, or aspect of self to the same extent as someone with intact awareness of their situation and predicament. No one would suggest the grief response occurs in coma or stuporous patients. However, most patients with aphasia are aware of their situation and predicament, suffer significant loss, and can be expected to experience the grief response due to the unwanted changes occurring to them.

Except for developmental loss, the onset of loss in each category is usually sudden. Sudden loss occurs without warning with little or no time to engage in preparatory grief. Before the loss, there may have been warnings that it was impending; however, the person may have been unaware of the signs because his or her attention may have been directed elsewhere.

TANGIBLE AND SYMBOLIC LOSSES

When an individual loses an object, person, or aspect of self, he or she is separated from the valued parts of life, and tries to either overcome the losses or accept them. This process occurs for real, tangible aspects of the losses, and for those aspects of life that have symbolic implications to the person.

The real, tangible losses can include people, abilities, and objects. They are discussed in detail below. Symbolic losses involve a person's self-concept. The symbolic aspects of the losses are related to the void and changes created in the person's self-concept. For example, a woman may lose her husband through death. The real, tangible loss results from the fact that he is no longer a part of her day-to-day life. His companionship, ideas, laughter, work products, and insights are lost forever. The woman's husband, and all of his exposure to her life, has been taken away by death. The tangible reality is that she is permanently separated from a loved and valued person. She no longer can touch or speak to him.

The symbolic realities of the loss involve the void and changes the woman must make in her self-concept because of her husband's death. She is now a widow. Not only has the woman lost her husband, she also has lost a part of herself. One of the losses involves her role as wife. Symbolically, the role may have supported her self-esteem. It may have provided a basis by which she defined important aspects of her life. More specifically, the woman's role of "wife to that particular husband" has been lost and never can be replaced. Even with a remarriage, she never can find a person identical to the one lost, nor can she recapture the essence of time and experience shared with the deceased man. The real loss of her husband combines with the symbolic losses experienced by the woman in the grief response.

A type of psychological separation similar to what occurs in aphasia happens when one party of a relationship persistently avoids or refuses intimate contact with another. Psychological separation usually precedes physical separation through divorce or departure. In marriage, when this happens, couples become disenchanted and avoid or refuse meaningful verbal or physical contact. The breakdown in communication further isolates the partners, and a spiral of negative emotions occur because of the persistent lack of communication and other factors. This perpetuates the psychological separation. Although there is some verbal and physical communication in psychological separation, it is superficial or meaningless and communication becomes ritualistic. When a partner in the marriage or relationship realizes the nature and extent of the psychological separation, the grief response can occur. Many individuals who have experienced divorce report that the "death" of the marriage occurred months, or even years, before the legal decree.

LOSS OF PERSON

Although a person with aphasia does not actually lose his or her loved ones, there can exist the sense of psychological separation discussed above due to the neurogenic communication disorder. Due to communication barriers, the patient may not be able to interact with loved ones as meaningfully, frequently, or easily as before. In patients with severe aphasia, especially those with comprehension deficits, the quality of social interaction with significant others can be substantially diminished. Even for patients with mild aphasia, the quality of the relationship with family members may be negatively affected. The sense of separation may be increased if patients are confined to long-term medical and rehabilitation facilities.

Grief can result from changes in living arrangements and relationships (Christ, Bonanno, Malkinson, and Rubin, 2003). The real loss of person includes physical separation from loved ones for long periods due to institutionalization, and is compounded by the communication barrier. There may also be the symbolic loss reported above. Symbolically, the patient and his family may see the neurogenic communication disorder as an insurmountable disability laying waste to what was previously a rich and rewarding relationship. Additionally, in some neurogenic communication disorders, there are sensory deficits which interfere with or prohibit intimate physical contact. In aphasia, the communication disorder crosses all language modalities, and consequently, also prohibits communication through reading, writing, and complex gestures.

For some patients, the onset of aphasia may exacerbate preexisting relationship problems. Problems with communication is the primary reason many marriages fail. For families having previous relationship problems, the communication disorder can perpetuate those troubles and worsen the relationship. The patient and his or her family's problems might not be fixable because they can no longer work through issues with communication.

Loss of person as a result of aphasia is both a stressor and barrier to adjusting to the disability. As discussed in Chapter 3, some aphasic disorders are associated with impaired defense mechanisms and coping styles, which reduce or eliminate the patient's ability to cope and adjust. Additionally, several psychological reactions and disorders discussed in Chapter 2, such as emotional lability, catastrophic reactions, perseveration, organic depression-anxiety, anosognosia, and homonymous hemianopsia can subject the patient to new and unusual stressors. Due to the communicative separation from loved ones, he or she is deprived of persons with whom he or she previously would analyze, discuss, and seek counsel about them.

Certainly, not all aphasias are of the severity to result in tangible and symbolic separation from loved ones. Some language disorders are mild with no appreciable reduction in the ability to functionally communicate. Others are temporary and patients make complete or near-complete recoveries. Never-the-less, many aphasias fundamentally disrupt the patients' ability to meaningfully relate to loved ones and impedes relationships with important people in their lives.

The role communication plays in maintaining significant relationships and developing new ones cannot be understated. Before the aphasia, the patient's relationships were created, nurtured and maintained by communication. Problems that surfaced were addressed primarily through verbal means. Speech and language served a means of sharing and venting emotions. Mutual problem-solving between the patient and his or her loved ones, especially in child-rearing and financial matters, were done verbally. Even for the person who was characteristically quiet and reserved, speech and language were vital and necessary aspects to the development and maintenance of human relationships. The onset of the aphasia removes or impairs an important element to human bonding. As discussed previously, the stroke, head trauma, or disease that causes the communication disorder also creates significant levels of stress for the patient. The more severe the communication disorder, the more extensive the disruption to the patient's relationships. The grief response results from the many changes occurring in interpersonal relationships. The relationship between the patient and his or her loved ones is altered significantly, and frequently irreversibly, by the neurogenic communication disorder. Although the patient has not lost his or her loved ones in a physical sense, he or she has lost the ability to communicate with them in a meaningful, purposeful, and constructive manner.

Case Studies, Illustrations, and Examples: Loss of Person

It was just one thing after another. You thought things would calm down now that the four children are grown and have their own families. You've put in your time. You and your wife took child-rearing seriously, and were communicative teammates during those stressful years. You planned, disagreed, argued, and considered every child-rearing option. There were the illnesses, the emergency room visits, broken bones, burns, and the sleepless nights of croup and teething. You attended every school meeting, concert, assembly, and participated in IEPs. You had the sex talks, and warned of the dangers lurking in the world. The teenage years were just about all you could handle what with the police knocking on the door and the experimentation with pot and booze. There were the scary motorcycle and car accidents. You shared their joy and angst of loves and loves lost. But now that you are "senior citizens," and you hate that label, you thought the stress and drama would end. All things considered, your children are doing fine and you are as proud as punch of each of them. Finally, you and your wife can relax and enjoy your golden years. Wrong again.

With social media, telephones, and texts, you still feel the stress and worry. Sadly, since your wife's stroke, you now go it alone. Her wise counsel is silenced by global aphasia. Now, you deal with difficult births, illnesses, separations, divorces, addictions, and accidents, not just of your children, but the grandchildren as well. And not surprisingly, the golden years are full of financial and health concerns for you and your teammate. You sorely miss your pre-stroke wife and the communication you once shared. Oh sure, she is still alive, and thank God for that, but she is a shell of what she once was. But, you soldier on, this time with your loving wife as an observer, and not the active participant you so depended on. At least, you have the memory of the rich relationship you once had and the communication that was its foundation and glue.

LOSS OF SOME ASPECT OF SELF

Loss of some aspect of self includes unwanted changes in health, body function, sense of worth, self-concept, family role, security, and perceived attractiveness. It occurs when a person is aware that she or he no longer possesses a previously normal and intact ability or function, and that the loss is irreversible. In patients with aphasia, loss of body function can occur with the ability to communicate, walk, and with several activities of daily living such as dressing, eating, and so forth.

The point at which a person becomes aware of the loss marks an important stage in acceptance of the disability. This is true in all dimensions, but it is particularly important in loss of self. As reported previously, the patient who has suffered traumatic head injury and resulting paralysis initially may not possess the perceptual and cognitive capabilities to understand the full extent of her or his impairments. However, as the patient's awareness returns, she or he will begin to have appreciation of what has been lost. Similarly, children with congenital disorders may never have been capable of unimpaired functioning, and only come to appreciate this fact later in childhood. The full realization that they are different and impaired in functioning may not occur until the child's perceptual skills, cognitive development, and experience permit it. There are two types of loss of self that are predominantly symbolic and there are few, if any, tangible aspects to them: loss of time and loss of innocence.

Loss of productive or meaningful use of time involves a person feeling that he or she has wasted part of his or her life. A person may feel that his or her youth was misspent or that a period of life devoted to learning was not spent as effectively as it should have been. People who obtain college degrees in professions to which they find they are unsuited may feel that they have wasted an important aspect of their lives. Time devoted to an unsuccessful marriage may make a person feel that they have squandered "the best part of life." Wasting of time has few tangible aspects to it. Loss of innocence, not just in the sexual realm, is another primarily symbolic loss. When a person realizes he or she no longer views the world with the innocence of a child, he or she may feel this as a serious loss. It is the loss of an innocent perspective on life. These predominantly symbolic losses are as irreversible and permanent as are losses in other dimensions. It is impossible to recapture time squandered and innocence lost.

The loss of language in aphasia can affect the patient's sense of self:

> It is possible to experience a sense of being that does not require language. But if a person's knowledge about his/herself is thrown into pure chaos the person may be in need of language to help construe the situation. In some way the aphasic person needs to have a working construct of 'before my illness' versus 'after my illness' and all its implications. Indeed, the grieving process can be viewed as making sense of the construct 'after my illness' and all its implications. (Brumfitt, 1996, p. 352)

Like loss of person, loss of self can have symbolic implications (Thompson and Mckeever, 2012). For example, loss of the ability to walk includes the physical limitations associated with mobility, but also greater implications such as lack of freedom and being unable to "stand on one's own two feet." The patient may feel that he or she is relegated to the status of a child because of permanent and irreversible physical losses, and is now a dependent ward of his or her family or institution. Brumfitt (1996) noted that aphasic patients may sense the loss of continuity with the past. They may perceive that independence and mobility are things of days-gone-by.

Loss of security is the loss of the predictability of usual reinforcements. Security simply means that the individual knows what to expect. Interestingly, people can be subjected to much negativity and consequently be unhappy, but there will be security even in this less-than-desirable predicament. People experience insecurity because of factors they cannot control. The loss of predictability of usual rewards or punishments means that the patient does not know what attitudes, behaviors, and thoughts will result in external or internal rewards, or which ones will result in punishments. The rules of the game have changed.

Some events clearly reduce the predictability of the usual rewards and punishments. One of the most significant events is the trauma associated with neurogenic communication disorders. Other events accompanying high levels of insecurity include marriage, the birth of a child, a new job, moving to a new community, attending college, retirement, and divorce.

The patient with aphasia is prone to a lack of security as a direct result of both the brain damage, and his or her awareness that life as he or she has known it is not likely to continue. In addition, there is the real threat of more devastating neurological impairments or death. Institutionalization itself creates insecurity regarding new routines and rehabilitation responsibilities. There is also the lack of security associated with financial responsibility for necessary medical care. The patient knows that health care services and institutionalization are expensive and can drain the family's resources. With many patients, there is a loss of security and the predictability of usual rewards and punishments. On some level, the patient realizes that the life he or she has known is unlikely to continue, and that there is the real threat of another stroke or other devastating medical incident occuring.

The tangible and symbolic aspects of loss of the ability to communicate are varied and many. To speak is to be potent. To be deprived of this fundamental ability reduces the individual to near-primitive levels of existence. Drives and wishes go unanswered. Expressions of emotions are reduced to the nonverbal mode, often leaving the listener confused. Life for the patient with aphasia can become an exercise in futility of expression, and an awkward game of charades. Indeed, the tangible and symbolic effects of aphasia can be profound and dramatically affect a person's quality-of-life.

Case Studies, Illustrations, and Examples: Loss of Self

So many things you took for granted. So many things came so easily. So many things were automatic, so you never gave them a second thought. But no more, since the stroke and aphasia changed all of that.

As you lie in bed with that sharp pain cutting through your back and stabbing at your leg, you try to roll onto your side. For decades, changing position remedied the discomfort and enabled you to go back to sleep. Sure, it was an irritant to your wife who complained you tossed and turned too much, but it worked. You and she managed to live with your back injury. But now things have changed.

You try and try to roll onto your side, but your efforts are to no avail. The muscles on your right side simply will not allow the transition. But the pain is still there, and growing with each minute as you lie in that uncomfortable position. Sadly, now you sleep alone in this nursing home bed, but at least you are not disturbing your wife. You try to press the button that will bring some kind of nurse or nurse's aide to your rescue and end the pain, but that too is unsuccessful. The blue button is out of your reach. "Help me," you attempt to shout, but no words come to mind and no sounds leave your mouth. The pain is becoming unbearable. Again, you try to shout "Help me," and again the room is silent. The words and actions that have been time-tested to end your pain have been lost to the stroke and aphasia. You lie back, enduring the pain, and try to accept your new lot in life.

LOSS OF OBJECT

Loss of object includes virtually any external object a person has come to value. The objects people value are highly variable and include homes, cars, pets, gardens, libraries, computers, recreation vehicles, and other things. One person may place a high value on his or her home, another on a rock collection, a cherished pet, and yet another on a vintage hot rod. Loss of the valued object has both real and symbolic implications to the person. Valued objects are lost to patients with aphasia because of physical and cognitive limitations and disabilities. For example, a patient may lose a recreation vehicle because he or she may be unable to drive, or the ability to garden because of confinement to a wheelchair. The motor home may have symbolic value to the person as a representation of the golden years of retirement, and gardening as a productive use of leisure time. Placement in a long-term medical care facility can cause separation from many valued objects, especially the patient's home and all of the valued objects in it. White (2001, p. 309) observes that the significance of the lost object to the individual determines the nature of the grief response: "For instance, an individual who loses a family heirloom in a fire may react not only to the lost financial value of the piece, but also to the lost sense of history and heritage that the piece represented."

Loss of objects can encompass the intangible. People can be expected to experience grief over loss of culture, power, religion, position in a company, and other statuses and beliefs. A patient may lose religious objects when he or she is separated from his or her church. For religious people, being unable to attend church regularly and participate in its rituals can be a significant negative consequence of neurological injury. Many religious ceremonies require functional communication abilities, and aphasia can interfere or eliminate a patient's ability to understand and participate in them. There is also the loss of symbols associated with a patient's religion. He or she can be denied the comfort and support they provide. Lost objects create significant voids in a patient's life, and the communication disorder can prevent or impair his or her ability to report the nature of the feelings associated with the losses.

Case Studies, Illustrations, and Examples: Loss of Object

Murphy had been a roofer all his working life. He started as a helper, and soon became supervisor of a roofing crew. Roofing is hard and dangerous work, and he resented the framers calling him and his crew "roof monkeys." Although decades ago he stopped using a roofing hammer and began using a pneumatic one, it still took a lot of energy to replace roof shingles. It is dangerous work, especially on homes and commercial buildings with steep roofs. More than one of his coworkers had slipped and nearly fallen to their injury or even death. They were saved by the safety harnesses the company required all roofers to wear. Murphy's twenty-five years as a roofer were sometimes pleasant, especially when the weather was good, but awful during the snow, wind, and rain. As he approached retirement, he knew he had put in his time as a roofer and was happy to give it up.

He and his wife patiently awaited retirement and eagerly anticipated the adventure of traveling the country in their brand new–at least to them–pre-owned Bounder motor home. Every chance he got, Murphy prepped the motor home for the lengthy road trips they would take. Sometimes, he would just sit in the driver's seat and fantasize about the states they would visit; their goal was to visit 49 of them. The Bounder was a fantastic machine, and a symbol of what would be his golden years: full of free time, leisure, adventure, quality time with his wife, and no more backbreaking physical labor.

But sadly, two weeks before his retirement, Murphy suffered a stroke and global aphasia. Now, as he sits in a wheelchair at the dining room table looking at the Bounder sitting idly in their backyard, and he feels a deep sense of loss. There will be no great adventures, no carefree time spent with his wife, no golden years envisioned. On some level, Murphy knows he has been robbed of his just rewards and the Bounder is a constant reminder of what the stroke has taken.

ACCEPTING UNWANTED CHANGE

The grief response is a collection of psychological adjustments a person makes to being permanently separated from something or someone of value. The first and most widely accepted grief model was proposed by Dr. Elizabeth Kübler-Ross (1969) in her landmark book: *On Death and Dying*. Kübler-Ross proposed five stages of the grieving process: denial, anger, bargaining, depression, and acceptance. While widely praised as a major advancement in the field of psychiatry, Kübler-Ross's model has been criticized particularly concerning the order of the stages leading to acceptance. Critics note that not everyone goes through all the stages, and some grieving persons go back and forth between different stages. Actually, Kübler-Ross addressed the order and sequence of the grieving process in her early writings on the subject and noted that the stages and progression are highly variable (Kübler-Ross, 1969; Kübler-Ross and Kessler, 2005).

The application of the grief model to the losses experienced by patients with aphasia is also controversial. Tanner (1980) first proposed the phase model of grief and its application to persons with communication disorders. Tanner and Gerstenberger (1988; 1996) applied the grief model to persons with aphasia. Parr, Byng, Gilpin, and Ireland (1997) examined the grief model concerning aphasic patients using an interview format. They found identifiable stages in aphasic patients, but no specific grieving progression through them. According to Lyon and Shadden (2001, p. 302):

> Thus, for a majority of Parr et al.'s subjects, there was no evidence of a set coping progression, although anger and denial were typically more prevalent at first, often giving way overtime to some form of internal compromise and/or acceptance. More characteristic, though, was a continuous and overlapping ebb and flow of all of Kübler-Ross's stages, their appearance and reappearance depending on the personal and collective subtleties of those affected.

The basic principle of the grief response model is that people with aphasia, like all humans when confronted with losses, go through a process of denial, frustrating attempts to overcome them, depressing awareness of their permanence, finality, irreversibility, and finally acceptance and resolution of the unwanted changes in their lives. Horn, Crews, Guryan, and Katsilometes (2016) report that given the unique needs of aphasia patients, creative approaches are necessary to address loss and grief issues.

THE ROAD TO ACCEPTANCE

Although there are several approaches to viewing the way patients with aphasia reach acceptance of unwanted changes in their lives, a phase model is useful in describing the grieving process (Boyd, 1998). The phase model is applicable to aware patients with significant and irreversible neurogenic communication disorders with the understanding that not all patients experience all the stages nor is there always a predictable progression through them. Additionally, in many patients, and their families, friends, and others, there are intermittent bouts of frustration involving anger. "For example, one person with aphasia might be 'angry' over the inability to work, 'in denial' about returning to pre-stroke communication levels, and 'accepting' that conversation with family and friends was impractical at the moment" (Lyon and Shadden, 2001, p. 301).

With respect to irreversible neurogenic communication disorders, there are several reactions a person may have to loss. The patient with a significant irreversible loss of language, who has the cognitive and perceptual capabilities to be aware of it, will experience denial, frustration, depression, and acceptance. Of course, the patient must have valued that which was lost. The order of occurrence of the reactions may vary, and the time spent in a stage may be prolonged or brief. Losses in each dimension can result in the reactions. They may occur independently of one another, or be present in such a way as to leave the person reacting to "loss in general" where the patient does not separate them, but feels the sense of loss as an overwhelming emotion. Each reaction will be discussed separately in their usual order of occurrence.

GRIEVING DENIAL

As noted above, patients with aphasia are likely to experience denial when first confronted with irreversible loss of person, some aspect of self, and objects. Denial is an early reaction to the loss, although the patient may be only partially aware of its irreversibility and permanence. It often occurs initially in the grief response, but can resurface throughout the course of grieving (Parr et al., 1997). Some patients may never experience denial, and others may chronically engage in it.

Freud (1961) considered denial as a defense mechanism to protect the ego, and Kübler-Ross (1969) found it to be an early response to loss. Denial is a stage of shock, disbelief, and incredulity. In denial, the patient may disbelieve what has happened and have an inability to comprehend the implications for his or her life. This defense mechanism and coping style can be characterized by the verbal report, "I do not believe it," made by individuals when initially confronted with the loss of a loved one. Tanner and Gerstenberger (1996; 1988) propose four themes of denial in the grief response from a psychiatric perspective: complete, partial, passive and mystical, and existential. It should be noted that denial is considered "generic" and underlies many of the other defense mechanisms and coping styles. These denial themes may be integral to several other psychological defense mechanisms and coping styles, and basically involves refusal to accept all or part of reality.

In complete denial, the patient believes he or she does not have a disability and often projects the communication disorder onto listeners. The patient believes that he or she is talking normally and the communication problems are the result of the listener's inability or unwillingness to understand his or her perfectly normal speech. This type of denial is frequently seen in jargon aphasic patients (Weinstein and Puig-Antich, 1974; Weinstein, Lyerly, Cole, and Ozer, 1966). As discussed in Chapter 2, denial is associated with specific brain lesions, but it is also at least partially related to the patient's need to protect his or her ego from anxiety and awareness of grievous losses. This statement summarizes complete denial and projection from the perspective of the patient: "I do not have a speech-language disorder and the communication problem is the result of the listener's inability or unwillingness to understand my perfectly normal speech."

Patients in partial denial may have awareness of some aspect of loss, but deny others. For example, a patient may be aware of loss of self concerning the ability to speak, but denies the implications of impaired communication in his or her relationships. Patients may also minimize the losses, believe they are temporary, or otherwise deny the totality of what has happened to them. Partial denial from the perspective of the patient can be summarized by this statement: "I have a communication disorder, but it is minor, temporary, and/or insignificant."

Patients with an external frame of reference may present with denial having a passive and mystical theme. The patient is at least partially aware that he or she has a communication disorder, but is certain that external forces will help with a complete recovery. The patient denies the reality of the communication disorder, and is usually passive about rehabilitation. He or she may direct his or her energies into prayer and faith healing rituals. "I have a significant neurogenic communication disorder, but it is temporary and God will make me whole again" summarizes the patient with a passive and mystical denial theme.

In contrast to patients with an external frame of reference, denial with an existential theme involves a person's belief in the ability to overcome aphasia through will and determination. These patients have an internal frame of reference. LaPointe (1997) found that patients who have an internal locus of control do better with adjustment to aphasia. Denial with an existential theme is only partial because the patient acknowledges the neurogenic communication disorder, but is unrealistic about his or her ability to overcome it. This statement summarizes denial with an existential theme: "I have a neurogenic communication disorder, but through my will and determination, I will overcome it and return to complete normalcy."

Denial is a lower order defense mechanism and coping style not requiring language, and is readily available to aphasic patients. Denial should be distinguished from misinformation. A patient in denial has been provided with accurate and complete information about the neurogenic communication disorder, yet denies all or part of it. The misinformed patient has not been accurately and completely apprised of his or her predicament. No matter the theme of the denial, it serves to prevent anxiety and buffer psychological pain. Denial permits the patient to avoid confrontation with the losses associated with the neurogenic communication disorder. In many cases, denial as an unrealistic positive view about disabilities can be congruent with mental health (Telford, Kralik, and Koch, 2005). At the very least, it allows the patient the time and opportunity to mobilize less radical defenses.

Confronting the patient with the losses associated with aphasia may result in deeper and more persistent denial. It is an attempt by the patient to deal with the unexpected losses and to mobilize other less radical defenses. The patient who successfully passes through the denial stage will move into stages of partial acceptance more easily. As reported above, denial is an extreme defense mechanism and coping style requiring a great deal of psychological energy. A less radical buffer to psychological pain should replace it as soon as possible. Brutal confrontation of denial can push the patient, and his or her family and friends, deeper into it.

Three factors influence the rate and ease with which the patient passes through grieving denial. The first factor is how much he or she is told about the disorder. If the patient perceives the extent of his or her illness, but is told very little, successful mobilization of other defenses could be delayed. Another factor influencing adjustment in this stage is the time available for the patient to resolve denial. A patient may be aware of time constraints. If there is little time available to the patient, as is often seen with the terminally ill, passage through this stage and other stages is frequently more rapid than might otherwise be expected. However, the opposite also may hold true.

The final factor that may affect the patient's ability to move through denial is his or her character before the onset of the communication disorder. According to LaPointe (1997), favorable pre-injury personality tendencies having a positive influence on coping with neurogenic communication disorders include: adaptability, persistence, attentiveness, and pleasant and stable moods. The frequent use of denial throughout a person's life as a primary defense mechanism and coping style may suggest a strong learned behavior. The patient is likely to resort to this behavior as a means of coping with brain injury and subsequent communication disorders (Scott and Tanner, 1990). The past use of denial as a habitual method of coping increases the probability that denial will be a primary means of adjustment to the communication disorder and related losses.

RESPONSE TO FRUSTRATION

Many patients with aphasia are frustrated by their attempts to overcome their losses and anger and bargaining are natural, normal reactions to that frustration. Anger and bargaining are expected reactions on the part of the patient to the loss of control that arises from two sources. First, the patient is generally frustrated by the inability to alter the course of events leading to the losses and unwanted changes in his or her life. There are many unalterable realities surrounding the brain and nervous system damage, and the patient is frustrated by his or her inability to change or eliminate them. Second, the patient may be frustrated by the inability to communicate with others normally. Although some aphasias are not frustrating, many are. There can be frustration associated with auditory comprehension and word finding. Reading, writing, and simple arithmetic may also be significantly impaired rendering the patient frustratingly unable to perform them as he or she once did easily. The chronic inability to consummate the communication act can be extremely frustrating and anger-provoking for some patients.

The anger felt by many patients with aphasia can take several forms. Some patients are passive in their anger and express it by missing appointments (see passive-aggression defense mechanism and coping style), isolating themselves from others, refusing treatment, and so forth. Other patients express anger by striking out at health care professionals, family, and friends. Angry patients with functional speech may use profanity and denigrate others.

Nonverbal patients may inwardly direct anger and feel guilt for their predicament. Some authorities believe this inward direction of anger causes depression. Frustration leads to anger, and the inner direction of it can bring on depression in some patients.

Anger is a natural and normal reaction to the frustration associated with grievous losses. Consequently, in most situations, it should neither be punished nor discouraged. However, if the anger displayed by the patient is destructive to himself or herself, or to others, then intervention is necessary. It is important that the patient understand that it is not the expression of anger that is being discouraged, only the inappropriate manner in which negative emotions are being ventilated. Exercise and other strenuous activities are constructive methods of dealing with anger.

Bargaining, another reaction to frustration, is the attempt by the patient to reduce or delay the losses. The patient offers some good behavior, or seeks help from a higher power or authority, to reduce, postpone, or eliminate the unwanted changes in his or her life. Bargaining patients may do so with themselves, family members, and God, and it may also occur with health care professionals (Kübler-Ross and Kessler, 2005). In the bargain, the patient turns over the disorder to a higher power or authority. Similar to denial, bargaining allows the patient to postpone becoming completely aware of what has been taken from him or her.

While bargaining with health care professionals may be nonverbal, it can be summarized in this statement: "If I enthusiastically participate in rehabilitation, and do everything required of me, I will get complete return of my abilities." The patient focuses on complete recovery of lost abilities, and his or her frustration is reduced because he or she believes the bargain will work. A positive aspect of bargaining is that the patient may be highly motivated and responsive to rehabilitation. Of course, health care professionals should avoid being unrealistic with patients about the value and outcomes of therapeutic services, and in fact, it is unethical to do so. The patient may require more of himself or herself than is desirable and practical, and will ultimately be disappointed. In some instances, the patient may be fixated in bargaining and never reach acceptance of his or her losses.

Health care professionals can reduce the frustration patients experience about the unwanted changes occurring in their lives by providing them with as much control as possible. Many decisions made in rehabilitation for the patient can be made by them. For example, many patients can and should be active participants in setting treatment goals and the procedures used to obtain them. Most importantly to reducing frustration during therapies, patients should succeed more than they fail. Clinicians should carefully design treatments to ensure that unobtainable goals do not unnecessarily frustrate patients. Carefully redefining the steps necessary to achieve an objective can accomplish this. Additionally, each session should begin and end with successful performance by the patient.

For grieving patients who are frustrated by their neurogenic communication disorders, special efforts should be taken to reduce the inherent frustration associated with speech production. By word or deed, clinicians should communicate to these patients that they cannot "force" speech to be produced correctly. Trial and error strategies are the best methods for word finding and speech programming and execution. Particularly with motor aphasia, forcing speech increases propositionality which decreases the accuracy of motor speech programming. In addition, with most patients, speech "perfection" is an unnecessary and unobtainable goal. The inherent frustration in neurogenic communication disorders can be reduced by recognizing that speech production need not be perfect to consummate communication.

Sometimes patients with aphasia will attempt to communicate something apparently important to their family, friends, and health care professionals, but are impotent in doing so. These often become frustrating games of charades. In those incidences where it is clear that the patient's thoughts will not be forthcoming, listeners should minimize the frustration associated with the verbal impotence. This can be done by communicating to the patient that the listener considers the information important, but because of the frustrating impediment, it will be returned to at a later date. This strategy does not negate the importance of what the patient intends to say; it does however, bring an end to the frustrating attempt to communicate it, at least temporarily.

GRIEVING DEPRESSION

Grieving depression occurs in aphasic patients who are aware they have suffered significant and valued losses. It is a natural, predictable result of permanent separation from valued people, aspects of self, and objects. Patients with aphasia may become depressed when they no longer deny the losses, feel anger about them, or realize bargaining will no longer prevent them. During grieving depression, the patient appreciates the full value of what has been lost. Losses that are less significant to the patient will produce less depression than those losses that are of greater value. However, it should be remembered that what is a grievous loss for one person, may only be an inconvenience to another.

Although depression can occur at any stage in the grieving process and reappear throughout it, patients become depressed when all other attempts to overcome the losses have failed. The duration of normal grieving depression may range from only a few days to several months, and some patients may become chronically depressed. Bouts of grieving depression may be triggered by stimuli for months, or even years, after the losses occur.

Normal grieving depression is also associated with the chemical changes occurring in the brain described in Chapter 3, but it is reactive and proportional to the losses experienced by the patient. This type of depression is also dependent on the hemisphere, site, and size of the brain lesion. Grieving depression is not simply a biochemical deficiency inducing prolonged feelings of sadness, hopelessness, anxiety, and helplessness. Of course, both organic and reactive depression may occur in some patients.

> Early on, for example, structural neurobiochemical changes within the brain, depending on the size and location of lesion, may dominate emotional stability. Later on, when the biochemistry of the brain has either stabilized or been augmented through antidepressant medications, reactive 'blues' in response to lasting functional losses may emerge as more influential. (Lyon and Shadden, 2001, p. 302)

Loneliness is particularly common in the severely impaired patient with aphasia due to the lack of ability to communicate verbally with staff, family, and friends (Tanner, Gerstenberger, and Keller, 1989). If the depression follows a period of bargaining and high levels of cooperation in rehabilitation, during depression, there may be a dramatic drop in the patient's motivation levels. Caregivers can also experience grieving depression. Studies show that family members report more negative emotions in stroke patients than self-reported by the patients, and aphasic patients tend to show little concern about or awareness of caregiver depression (Lyon and Shadden, 2001).

Grieving depression may also be psychotic and accompanied by mania and agitation (Tanner and Gerstenberger, 1989, 1996). These psychotic episodes may be the result of the patient returning to denial. "Persistent euphoria and mania, however, signal regression to radical defenses and/or psycho-organic deficits symptomatic of psychotic depression" (Tanner and Gerstenberger, 1996, p. 317). Grieving depression should not be considered abnormal, since it is appropriate to the losses experienced by the patient with aphasia. "Treating depression is a balancing act. We must accept sadness as an appropriate, natural stage of loss without letting an unmanaged, ongoing depression leach our quality of life" (Kübler-Ross and Kessler, 2005, p. 23).

The overall suicide rate is 10.9 deaths per 100,000 people (National Institute of Mental Health, 2007). However, some authorities believe this is a low estimate due to under-reporting, and it does not account for the many depressed people who attempt suicide. In grieving depression, suicide is the result of the patient wanting to avoid and escape the realities of the loss and the depression. According to the National Institute of Mental Health (2007), the suicide rate is higher in the elderly. Due to the higher risk of suicide, clinicians should be alert to signs of it, including a family history of suicide, reports, and previous attempts.

RESOLUTION AND ACCEPTANCE

The goal of the grief response is resolution and acceptance of the losses. Usually acceptance is the final stage of the grieving process, but it may be partial or complete. A patient may be accepting about one aspect of the losses he or she has suffered, but not accepting of another (Lyon and Shadden, 2001). Additionally, some accepting patients may return to previous aspects of the grief response when triggered by stimuli or general stress.

Acceptance is not the same as resignation to the losses suffered by the patient with aphasia. Resignation implies that the patient tolerates the losses and the despair associated with them. In resignation, the patient psychologically surrenders to the unwanted changes in his or her life. Resignation to the losses is reflected in this statement: "I have suffered terrible losses, but there is nothing I can do about the situation, so I will tolerate them." Resolution and acceptance, on the other hand, means the patient feels neither good nor bad about what has been lost and he or she is often void of emotions about them. In resolution and acceptance, the patient has assimilated the losses into a larger psychological framework.

Patients with aphasia who have resolved and accepted their losses remain good rehabilitation candidates. In fact, many patients are more realistically motivated to improve their communication abilities and have more energy to do so. They can redirect their energies to rehabilitation because they are no longer attempting to psychologically prevent their losses and are no longer depressed. They continue to strive for improvement.

> Treatments for the consequences of aphasia's chronicity are only in their infancy, and are diverse in their form, purpose, setting, and type of participation. It seems likely that we will find that no single means of management, (group, dyadic, or individual) or single participant (person with aphasia, significant other, family, friend, employer, or stranger) is sufficient to return disrupted life systems to preferred or optimal states of wellness. (Lyon and Shadden, 2001 p. 304)

Case Studies, Illustrations, and Examples: The Grief Response

Card playing has always been therapeutic for you. From gin to solitaire, there is something calming about shuffling, dealing, holding, and handling cards. Even when you were too young to play serious card games, you would lie next to that big old fireplace on cold winter nights and make houses out of them. Some card houses would have two or three stories and only your carelessness, or your big brother's meanness, would cause them to tumble to the carpet. You have always been able to lose yourself in Jacks, Kings, deuces, and eights.

You especially love poker. Growing up, you would read about the great card players of the West: Doc Holiday, Bat Masterson, and Wyatt Earp. Maverick was your favorite television show and Bret, not Bart, was the best poker player of them all.

In college, the weekly poker game was your favorite outlet, and you might modestly say, a good source of income. Early on, you learned to keep your beer consumption to a minimum and let the others make foolish, costly mistakes, like drawing to an inside straight. For years before entering the nursing home, you would have weekly poker games with your friends from work. Each player would bring chips, nuts, crackers, and beer. Ah, the smell of a cigar still returns you to those wonderful evenings of boasts, bluffs, and bets. Even now, sitting at this card table with quad canes, walkers, and wheelchairs parked next to it, you still love a good game of poker. Lately, though, it seems the stakes have been getting higher.

Your stroke happened eight months ago. It was the darndest thing. You had just gotten up and were opening a new can of coffee when your right hand wouldn't twist the can opener. Then, in a flash, your whole right side gave way. Thank goodness, your fall to the floor alerted Terry. You don't remember the ambulance ride to the hospital, or the hours spent in the emergency ward. Nor, do you remember the worried looks on your children's faces or the loving hugs of your grandchildren. For weeks, you were in an oxygen starved netherworld, partially knowing what had happened and partially, wonderfully, oblivious to the terrible event that had taken so much from you.

During your stint in the rehabilitation unit, you started having flashes of awareness of all that had been taken by the stroke. You couldn't walk, even if you could get out of bed by yourself. Eating was done with the assistance of a nurse's aide. And oh, the indignities of being unable to get to and from the toilet without help. Stuck in the hospital, you were separated from your home, car, kitchen, and weekly poker nights. You missed the security of routines, your dog Maggie, and your evening walks with the crisp crunching snow beneath your shoes. You sorely missed the little things; those nightly walks, your dog, and the white vapor rising from your lips.

But the stroke has taken far more than your balance, poker nights, and walks. It has taken your loved ones. Oh sure, Terry, the kids, and grandchildren are still physically there. They were not taken from you by death. But, because you can't communicate, your life with them has been reduced to the basics. You want to talk to them about the big issues, the costs, the options, the future, but the bridge of communication has collapsed. You reach out for meaning in those relationships, but are thwarted by verbal impotence.

Your life has changed, and as time marches on, you realize many of the changes are permanent. Even though you regained some abilities to walk and talk, the unwanted realities of life after stroke persist. There is now a great distance between you and the people and things you so cherished. Like losing the big pot in poker, the stroke has taken your life's winnings.

The burden of losing so much, so fast, is buffeted by your mind's defenses. Just beyond the senses, your mind blocks the painful realities of loss. There are minutes, and even hours, where you are oblivious of your plight. In denial, you find relief from the pain of loss. You have brief periods of respite where the sad reality of loss is gone. You hide in the corner of denial, buffeted from the all-encompassing pain of loss. Denial is like a protective door allowing reality to enter gradually and slowly, and when you deem the time is right.

The frustration of your predicament causes anger to rear its ugly head. You have been dealt a bad hand, and there are no more draws. You would like to change the reality of the situation, but on a deeper level, you know that is impossible. It angers you that you cannot do the things which once came easily. It angers you that your loved ones are unreachable, like some large cavern separates you. It angers you that Maggie walks alone at night.

Perhaps, you bargain, if you work hard in therapy, or find a "miracle" therapist, doctor, or drug, your life will return to normal. You pray for help, offer a vice for a reprieve from these losses, but even prayer has been taken by the communication disorder. The intimate words shared between you and God have been taken by the devil stroke.

You finally give up trying to overcome the losses. It's futile. The denial no longer buffers the pain, the anger serves no purpose, and there are no bargains to be struck. The cards have all been turned over, and you have lost the hand. The pot of life's valuables no longer belongs to you. Ironically, you feel the full value of that which was lost as the depression overwhelms you.

The depression you feel is not the result of chemicals gone awry in your brain. The depression you feel is grief. Humans are no stranger to it; it has been in the cards since the beginning, but that knowledge doesn't help reduce your pain. You fall into lethargy and sadness preoccupied with thoughts of those beloved people, things, and abilities which have been taken from you. Thoughts of death, dying, and loss saturate your heart and mind. You wonder about the meaning of it all.

The pain of loss gradually subsides. One afternoon, you realize that hours have gone by without the pain of grief. Hours of calm acceptance gradually become days and weeks. You soon realize that acceptance is not the same as resignation. In resignation, you only tolerate what has been taken from you. In acceptance, you understand the losses in the scheme of things; a scheme of which you are a part. Loss was always in the cards, and there would be no excitement in poker without it. You know that there would never be the joy of a royal flush without the sorrow of two, three, four, five, seven. You find yourself basking in the pleasure of knowing what you had, rather than saddened by the passing of it.

The steps in reaching acceptance were not smooth, nor did you not backslide. Some steps were brief and almost skipped, while others made it seem like you had feet of clay. Your difficult journey to acceptance was helped by your friends and loved ones. It seems that people just naturally know what to do. After all, loss has been around forever, and so too has the compassionate human spirit.

As you watch the cards being dealt for the last hand of the night, you realize that your life has not really been a gamble. Poker is not a metaphor for life. In poker, the outcome is unknown and determined by skill, luck, and chance. In life, loving and losing were determined long before your consciousness arose from matter and energy. Life is not a game of Texas Hold-Em, and nothing was ever more certain than love and loss. It was just a matter of that persistent illusion called "time."

HEALTH CARE PROFESSIONALS AND THE GRIEVING PATIENT

There are several factors that affect the normal grieving process and many of them can be influenced by the clinician. Health care professionals enter aphasic patients and their families lives at a difficult time. Although there is little that can be done to prevent the losses which have happened to the patient, thoughtful, caring clinicians can say and do things that can help the patient reach acceptance of them. With patients who have experienced irreversible losses, the clinician's actions can be positive and assist in reducing the person's psychological pain. There are also actions and statements that can interrupt the process of accepting the disorder and its implications. The clinician should do all he or she can to produce an environment that is conducive to rapidly moving through the grieving process. This may also involve enlisting the assistance of family and friends in approaching the patient in the proper way. The patient's family members are important members of the rehabilitation team and they should be aware of the way people reach acceptance of unwanted change (Tanner, 2008). Below are strategies used by the clinician to help the patient move through the grieving process to ultimately reach acceptance of his or her real and symbolic losses (Table 4-1).

Avoid Rewarding Denial

Rewarding denial can interrupt the course of the grieving process. Although it is helpful to a certain extent, denial is an extreme psychological defense and should be replaced as soon as possible by less radical buffers to psychological pain. It is important to pass through all the stages of

TABLE 4-1
FACILITATING THE GRIEVING PROCESS IN APHASIA

DO	DON'T
1. Permit the patient control	1. Reward denial
2. Provide the patient with a realistic perspective	2. Contribute to frustration
	3. Bargain with the patient
3. Acknowledge the reality of the losses	4. Provide secondary gains
4. Listen	5. Provide early distraction
	6. Interrupt private grief

the grieving process, though brief some may be, and it is not to the patient's advantage to state or reinforce untruthful remarks. Of course, brutal confrontation of the reality of the losses should be avoided. The goal is to be open, honest, and tactful.

Denial is a necessary and productive stage to the grieving process, and the clinician should not attempt to shake the patient from it. As discussed previously, brutal confrontation of denial may push the patient deeper into it. Most patients move naturally from denial to more productive stages when their needs dictate it.

All patients should be left with a degree of hope. Hope is necessary to mental health, and to optimal recovery. If a patient, or his or her family and friends, ask for a prognosis from the clinician, the probabilities method of stating it can indicate a realistic potential for recovery without eliminating hope. By avoiding the extreme percentages, such as 0% or 100%, the clinician can provide a prognosis without causing despair. Even a 10% probability of recovery offers something for which to strive and hope. The probabilities method of stating prognosis also gives the clinician necessary latitude for error. No one can be 100% certain that a patient will or will not recover his or her speech and language abilities. After providing a prognosis, the clinician should allow time for counseling and emotional support. If the patient, or his or her family, clings to unrealistic beliefs, referral to a counselor, psychologist, or psychiatrist is warranted.

Avoid Contributing to Frustration

The patient with irreversible losses experiences frustration that causes anger and bargaining. The patient is frustrated by his or her attempts to overcome the loss, and tries to defend against it. Frustration, and all manifestations of it, are natural and expected aspects of the grief response.

The anger expressed by the frustrated patient can take many forms. Some patients display passive anger by refusing therapy or by isolating themselves. Severely involved patients can overtly express anger by throwing things, hitting others, or using obscene gestures. Less severely involved patients may call people ugly names or use profanity in an attempt to cope with the frustration. As noted in previous sections many patients with aphasia direct their anger inward. Patients with severe communication disorders are prone to inner direction of anger because they cannot verbally express themselves. Premorbidly, patients prone to inner direction of anger typically were verbal in their anger response.

Rarely should anger be punished or even discouraged. First, anger is an expression of feelings. As such, even in its raw forms, it is communication. For the severely involved patient, it may be one of the few feelings that can be expressed. Second, anger is a natural consequence of frustration and should be recognized as an important part of the grieving process. Acceptance of the patient and his or her predicament by family, friends, and health care professionals includes acceptance of the person's emotions. The patient's anger should be understood rather than reacted to by clinicians and family.

It is also important to understand that not all anger is a result of the patient's losses. All anger is not a part of grieving. Anger can be caused by insensitive family, friends, and health care professionals. Those around the patient should seek the cause of the anger and not automatically assume that it is a result of the frustration associated with the losses. "The best way to diffuse hostility is to diagnose its cause and then target your intervention accordingly" (Carlat, 1999, p. 48). Telford, Kralik, and Koch (2005) note that health care professionals who adopt the stage theory of grieving may not attentively listen when patients with chronic illnesses relate their unique stories about coping with their illnesses.

Obviously, not all displays of anger are acceptable, constructive reactions by the patient. There are times when displays of anger should be discouraged. When the expression of anger is destructive to the patient, other persons, or a facility, intervention is required. This can be done in several ways.

First, the clinician should be careful in stressing that it is not the anger that is being discouraged, but the negative manner in which the patient is expressing it. Explaining this to a patient with severely impaired receptive abilities may be a challenge. Second, attempts should be taken to redirect the patient's anger. For example, the patient should be provided with a harmless object which can be used for emotional ventilation. Also, it is not disastrous to a medical facility if a food tray is thrown to the floor by an angry patient. Neither is it disastrous if a chair is turned upside down because of the patient's frustration. Placed in the proper perspective, these acts are insignificant given the profound changes that have occurred to the patient. Allowing the patient to slap his or her hand on a table is an example of a relatively safe redirection of anger. If redirection of anger is impossible or impractical, the third approach involves restraints or punishment of destructive acts. Verbal punishment or withholding of pleasurable activities can be used in a program of behavior management. The least desirable alternative is the use of restraints although sometimes they are necessary.

As reported above, bargaining, another manifestation of frustration, is a natural and necessary part of the grieving process; however, excessive bargaining can be problematic. Hope is an essential element to acceptance, but unrealistic hope should be avoided. As reported previously, patients in the bargaining stage tend to be very motivated in therapies. This is especially true when bargaining occurs with health care professionals. The clinician can unintentionally provide false hope and perpetuate the unrealistic bargain because of what is said and not said. The clinician wants the patient to make maximum progress, and it is natural to avoid saying anything that will reduce the patient's motivation. It is difficult for the clinician to suggest that the patient's efforts in therapy probably will not result in complete recovery. There is the realistic fear that the patient will give up. Some patients do lose motivation when the bargain with the clinician is found to be unrealistic. Although bargaining with the patient may produce positive short-term results, the long-term effects may interrupt the necessary grief work. Some people fixate in bargaining and never reach an acceptance of loss. Patients in the bargaining stage often require more of themselves than is practical or desirable. In cases where complete recovery from neurogenic communication disorders is not probable, the clinician should counsel the patient to be realistic, yet optimistic.

A certain amount of frustration experienced by the grieving patient can be eliminated by the clinician. Sensitive therapists can structure the patient's activities to eliminate many unnecessary obstacles. As a rule in therapy, the patient should succeed more than he or she fails. The patient should be kept on a level of success that results in improvement. When a patient persistently fails at an activity, it is not his or her fault; it is an error in clinical judgment on the part of the therapist. The clinician needs to redefine the steps necessary to achieve the goals.

One of the first statements which should be made to the patient with a neurogenic communication disorder is: "You cannot force the word or utterance out." This needs to be communicated to the patient, by whatever means possible, early on. Easy trial and error succeeds at speech, whereas forcing the utterance or word results in increased frustration, anxiety, anger, and depression. When a patient continues to try to communicate something, but is unsuccessful, the clinician should defuse the situation. As reported previously, this can be done by saying, "I don't understand now, we'll come back to it later." This acknowledges the importance of the patient's thought, but does not allow the frustration to continue.

Avoid Providing Secondary Gains

People empathize with the pain experienced by the bereaved. As a result, an individual in the grieving process may receive more attention, sympathy, and contact with others than he or she normally would receive. The support provided by friends and relatives is important to minimizing the pain experienced by the griever and, as a rule, it should not be discouraged. However, sometimes that attention, sympathy, and contact provided by others meet secondary needs in the griever. There can be secondary gains provided by the loss, and it may be difficult for the individual to give up the role of griever.

Lonely patients, especially those confined to a nursing home, may receive secondary gains. They receive attention from clinicians on a regular basis, and unfortunately, for some patients, this may be the only outside visitors they get. Sometimes, this contact with a kind, caring person can result in interruption of the grieving process and less progress in speech and language recovery than otherwise would be possible because of secondary gains. Clinicians should be careful not to create emotional dependency.

Avoid Heavily Sedating Drugs

Most physicians appreciate information from health care professionals about the nature and dosages of medications provided to rehabilitation patients. Many physicians recognize the value of the close relationship between the patient and therapist when assessing the effects of medication, especially in the psychological realm.

For the grieving patient, tranquilizers, sedatives, alcohol, and other drugs, should be avoided during the acute stages of the grieving process. Awareness of the loss is an important aspect of eventual acceptance of it. These drugs can interfere with the awareness phase, and they do not eliminate the emotional pain associated with loss, they only postpone it. Certainly, there are cases where medication is advisable and beneficial, but heavily sedating drugs to eliminate the grieving process is contraindicated. Medications cannot resolve a crisis but psychopharmacologic agents can help reduce its emotional intensity. They are beneficial when used temporarily or when other options are not available.

Emotional lability and grieving depression share common symptoms. Frequent and intense emotional outbursts may be indicative of persistent emotional lability (see Chapter 3), or unresolved loss and fixation in depression. With both disorders, an effective treatment may be mood elevating medications. However, even in these cases, the medications should be periodically reduced or removed to decide if the patient can regain emotional inhibition or reach an acceptance of the losses without them.

Avoid Interruption of Private Grief

Privacy is hard to come by in many medical care facilities. Most hospitals and nursing homes place two or more patients in a room. Additionally, some facilities either inundate the person with activities or totally neglect him or her. Both extremes should be avoided. The grieving patient should be provided with regular times and places where he or she can be alone. The patient needs time and opportunity to become aware of the losses and to work through them.

Sometimes, friends and relatives suggest that the person become immersed in work or hobby. The assumption is that the patient can attend to other activities, and thus forego the pain associated with the losses. During the later stages of the grieving process, these suggestions may be necessary and helpful, especially if the patient experiences fixations in any of the stages of the grief reaction. However, overindulgence in work or hobby during the early stages of the grief reaction may be counter-productive. The patient may avoid confrontation of the loss. Unhealthy early distractions can include moving to a new community, a new job, or the demands of an intensive rehabilitation program.

Permit the Patient Control

The psychological pain felt by a patient with aphasia during the grieving process is partially due to his or her impotency in altering the course of unwanted events that have led to the losses. The feelings of helplessness that accompany grieving can be reduced by allowing the patient to control certain aspects of his or her life. Lack of control in the patient's life contributes to frustration and anxiety about losses. The more control the patient is provided over his or her life, the less frustration he or she will experience.

In many medical care facilities, the staff dictates when the patient can engage in many day-to-day activities. The institution's routine reflects the staff's, not the patient's needs. The result is that many day-to-day activities of the institution are outside the patient's control. The patient must awaken at times demanded by the staff, eat when the tray arrives, and go to therapy when the schedule dictates. Even visiting hours are set by the facility. There is little the patient can do to control even the minor aspects of his or her life. The dehumanizing effects of rigidly adhering to others' schedules combine with the fact the patient is blocked in his or her efforts to stop the course of the losses. It is no wonder that many patients react with bargaining, rage, and depression.

Patients with communication disorders lack more control than do those with intact powers of speech and language. A verbal person can demand his or her rights, request privileges, and resist impositions. Often, a verbal person will get his or her way. Indeed, "the squeaky wheel gets the grease," but the patient with aphasia is often at a distinct disadvantage. Too often, the medical staff neglects to discuss with the speech and language disordered patient his or her preferences regarding facility routines.

The health care professional can be instrumental in providing the patient with control. She or he can also advocate for the patient with other members of the staff to create conditions where basic decisions can be made by the patient. It is not difficult to create an environment where the patient can make most of the decisions about his or her day-to-day activities. For example, the patient can be allowed to decide which room to use for therapy, or if therapy should be provided on a particular day. Higher functioning patients can decide what activities to emphasize in therapy and when to take breaks. The same principles can be applied to other therapies and nursing procedures. Medical care routines should reflect the patient's needs and not those of the institution.

Provide the Patient with Perspective

During the acute stages of the grieving process, the patient may feel that there will never be an end to the emotional pain over the losses. The patient may feel caught in a vicious cycle of loss and grief. During this time, the clinician can be of immense help to the bereaved by providing perspective regarding the eventual acceptance of the losses, and the reduction of sorrow that accompanies acceptance. By placing the loss in perspective, the clinician allows the patient to see the light at the end of the painful, grieving tunnel.

Perspective can be provided to the patient by telling him or her about the grieving process. The clinician should explain that the sorrow and pain will end. The process the patient is going through is one of healing. Counseling should be employed to help the patient realize the finite

Figure 4-1. Stages of resolution of loss in aphasia.

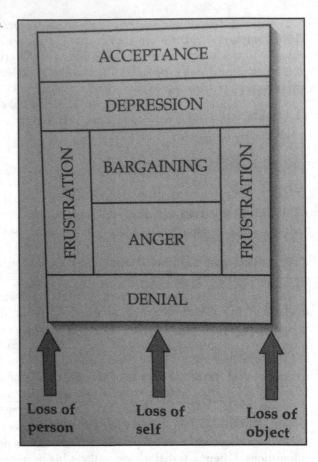

nature of grieving and to become aware, on a personal level, that the pain and sorrow will end. It can be comforting to a grieving person to have someone explain that there will be an end to the sorrow, and that life will have pleasures and joys in it again. However, communicating this to a patient with severe receptive language deficits is challenging. One way of doing this may be to provide examples of patients with severe aphasia who, by their manner, appear to be well-adjusted and accepting of their disability. Figure 4-1 shows the dimensions of loss and the stages many people with aphasia go through on the road to acceptance.

Acknowledge the Reality of the Loss

It is natural for the patient's family, friends, and health care professionals to want to avoid discussion of what has been lost. Some people believe that by changing the topic of conversation they are helping the griever. But when family, friends, and health care professionals avoid discussing the losses, they deprive the patient of necessary and productive expression of grief. To grieve properly, the patient must become aware of the losses and acknowledge the reality of them. In this process, the clinician can serve a very important function.

Unless the clinician has known the patient in the past, he or she is considered a detached observer concerning the losses. As a result, the patient may not feel the need to maintain a role and be inhibited in his or her emotional expressions when communicating with the clinician. For example, the patient with aphasia may also be a husband, father, grandfather, or friend, and because of these different roles, he may feel the responsibility to act in a particular way. The patient may not feel comfortable in expressing fear to his or her partner or children. Anger may not be expressed uninhibitedly to friends. The clinician, however, is devoid of many sensitive roles, and as such, the patient may feel less inhibited to express personal and complex emotions. The patient may be more open to a detached observer than he or she would be to loved ones.

When confronted with the grieving patient, some individuals feel the need to explain, defend or rationalize the losses, and this is not necessarily disruptive to the process of reaching acceptance. Many bereaved individuals welcome advice, suggestions, or philosophies of life presented in this way. However, silence is often very therapeutic, and it may be welcomed by the patient. He or she may just need someone who will listen.

Sometimes, people who encourage the patient to express the meaning of the losses will feel that a statement must be made which will "make it all right." Few people have this ability. There are no expressions that will permanently eliminate the pain felt by the bereaved. These attempts, however well-intentioned, are rarely appreciated by the patient and are often perceived as attempts to negate the losses or his or her feelings about them. It is also possible, that what is perceived as a positive statement may be inappropriate to the patient. Her or his beliefs may be different. People who have strong religious and philosophical values should avoid the assumption that the bereaved shares those views.

It is part of the clinician's responsibility to do all he or she can to facilitate the grieving process in patients with aphasia. Helping a patient accept loss is as much of a clinical responsibility as are the therapies. No matter the dimension of the loss, the clinician should regard the patient as in a period of significant change and transition. The goal of rehabilitation includes facilitation of the grieving process and ultimate acceptance of the losses by the patient and his or her family. The process of grieving helps the bereaved appreciate the true significance of the losses. With appropriate intervention, resolution of the losses can be a positive experience in growth and transformation.

CHAPTER SUMMARY

There comes a time when patients must cease attempting to overcome the aphasia and other related disorders and focus attention on resolving and accepting the permanent unwanted changes in their lives. Neurogenic communication disorders are associated with real and symbolic losses of people, aspects of self, and valued objects. Many patients experience grieving denial, frustration, grieving depression, and eventual resolution and acceptance of the losses they have experienced. While many patients pass through predictable stages leading to resolution and acceptance of the losses associated with neurogenic communication disorders, others have similar but relatively independent psychological reactions. Health care professionals can be important in facilitating the grieving process to help patients eventually resolve and accept their losses.

REFERENCES

American Psychiatric Association. (2013). *Diagnostic and statistical manual of mental disorders* (5th ed.). Arlington, VA: American Psychiatric Association.

Boyd, M. (1998). Theoretical basis of psychiatric nursing. In M. Boyd, & M. Nihart (Eds.), *Psychiatric nursing*. Philadelphia, PA: Lippincott, Williams & Wilkins.

Brumfitt, S. (1996). Losing your sense of self: What aphasia can do. In C. Code, & D. Muller (Eds.), *Forums in clinical aphasiology*. London, UK: Whurr.

Carlat, D. (1999). *The psychiatric interview*. Philadelphia, PA: Lippincott, Williams & Wilkins.

Christ, G., Bonanno, G., Malkinson, R., and Rubin, S. (2003). Bereavement experiences after the death of a child. In M. Field, & R. Behrman (Eds.), *When children die: Improving palliative and end-of-life care for children and their families* (pp.553-579). Washington, DC: National Academy Press.

Code, C., Hemsley, G., and Herrmann, M. (1999). The emotional impact of aphasia. *Seminars in speech and language, 20*(1), 19-31.

Freud, S. (1961). *The ego and the id: Standard edition of the complete psychological works of Freud*, Vol XIX. London, UK: Hogarth Press.

Horn, E., Crews, J., Guryan, B., and Katsilometes, B. (2016). Identifying and addressing grief and loss issues in a person with aphasia: A single-case study. *Journal of Counseling & Development, 94*(2), 225-233.

Kübler-Ross, E. (1969). *On death and dying.* New York, NY: Macmillan.

Kübler-Ross, E., and Kessler, D. (2005). *On grief & grieving.* New York, NY: Scribner.

LaPointe, L. (1997). Adaptation, accommodation, aristos. In L. LaPointe (Ed.), *Aphasia and related neurogenic language disorders* (2nd ed.). New York, NY: Thieme.

Lyon, J., and Shadden, B. (2001). Treating life consequences of aphasia's chronicity. In R. Chapey (Ed.), *Language intervention in aphasia and related neurogenic communication disorders* (4th ed.). Philadelphia, PA: Lippincott Williams and Wilkins.

National Institute of Mental Health (2007). Suicide in the U. S.: statistics and prevention. Retrieved from http://www.nimh.nih.gov/health/publications/suicide-in-the-us-statistics-and-prevention.shtml

Parr, S., Byng, S., Gilpin, S., and Ireland, C. (1997). *Talking about aphasia.* Philadelphia, PA: Open University Press.

Scott, K., and Tanner, D. (1990). *Recovery from brain insult: Investigation of patient adaptation and recovery.* Paper presented to the annual convention of the Canadian Association of Speech-Language Pathologists and Audiologists, Vancouver, BC.

Spillers, C. (2007, August). An existential framework for understanding the counseling needs of clients. *American Journal of Speech-Language Pathology, 16*(3), 191-197.

Tanner, D. (1980). Loss and grief: Implications for the speech-language pathologist and audiologist. *Journal of the American Speech and Hearing Association, 22,* 916-928.

Tanner, D. (2003, Winter). Eclectic perspectives on the psychology of aphasia. *Journal of Allied Health, 32*(4), 256-260.

Tanner, D. (2006). *Case studies in communication sciences and disorders.* Columbus, OH: Prentice-Hall/Merrill.

Tanner, D. (2007). *The medical-legal and forensic aspects of communication disorders, voice prints, and speaker profiling.* Tucson, AZ: Lawyers and Judges Publishing Company.

Tanner, D. (2008). *The family guide to surviving stroke and communication disorders* (2nd ed.). Boston, MA: Jones and Bartlett.

Tanner, D. (2009). *The psychology of neurogenic communication disorders: A primer for health care professionals.* New York, NY: iUniverse.

Tanner, D., and Gerstenberger, D. (1988). The grief response in neuropathologies of speech and language. *Aphasiology, 1*(6), 79-84.

Tanner, D., and Gerstenberger, D. (1989). *Psychological conflict and defense in aphasia.* A mini-seminar presented at the Annual Convention of the American-Speech-Language Hearing Association, St. Louis, MO.

Tanner, D., and Gerstenberger, D. (1996). Clinical forum 9: The grief model in aphasia. In C. Code, & D. Muller (Eds.), *Forums in clinical aphasiology* (pp. 313-318). London, UK: Whurr.

Tanner, D., Gerstenberger, D., and Keller, C. (1989). Guidelines for treatment of chronic depression in the aphasic patient. *Journal of Rehabilitation Nursing, 14*(2), 77-87.

Telford, K., Kralik, D., and Koch, T. (2005). Acceptance and denial: Implications for people adapting to chronic illness: Literature review. *Journal of Advanced Nursing 55*(4), 457-464.

Thompson, J., and Mckeever, M. (2012). The impact of stroke aphasia on health and well-being and appropriate nursing interventions: An exploration using the Theory of Human Scale Development. *Journal of Clinical Nursing, 23*(3-4), 410-420.

Weinstein, E., Lyerly, O., Cole, M., and Ozer, M. (1966). Meaning in Jargon Aphasia. *Cortex, 2*(2): 165-187.

Weinstein, E., and Puig-Antich, J. (1974). Jargon and its analogues. *Cortex, 10*(1), 75-83.

White, L. (2001). *Foundations of nursing: Caring for the whole person.* Albany, NY: Delmar Thompson Learning.

Glossary

A-: A prefix indicating the complete absence of function or ability.

Abstract attitude: Ability to symbolize and categorize verbal and nonverbal information; generalized ability to understand relationships.

Acalculia: The inability to perform and understand simple mathematics due to neurological injury.

Acceptance: In grieving, this is the final stage in the process of accepting unwanted change. Placing loss into a larger framework and being removed from emotional involvement.

Acquired aphasia: Loss of language occurring after birth as a result of disease or injury.

Agnosia: The inability to recognize and appreciate the significance of sensory stimuli; usually specific to one modality of communication.

Agrammatism: Loss of the ability to understand and use the grammar of a language. The omission of grammatical units of language.

Agraphia: The inability to write secondary to central language deficits and not due to limb paralysis; the inability to express oneself in writing.

Alexia: The inability to read not due to visual acuity deficits or blindness.

Altruism: Demonstration of concern for others.

Amnesia: Partial or complete inability to recognize or recall past events; loss of memory.

Tanner, D.C.
The Psychology of Aphasia: A Practical Guide for Health Care Professionals
(pp 103-114). © 2017 Taylor & Francis Group.

Aneurysm: A ballooning or swelling in the wall of an artery.

Anomia: Loss of the ability to recall words; not limited to nouns.

Anosognosia: The inability to perceive, recognize and accept body parts; denial of disability.

Anoxia: Lack of oxygen to the brain.

Anterograde amnesia: Loss of the ability to form, store, and recall new memories.

Anxiety: Worry, angst, fear, and apprehension. Lacking a sense of well-being, or in the extreme, a feeling of impending doom.

Aphasia: Multimodality inability to encode, decode, and/or manipulate symbols for the purposes of verbal thought or communication; the loss of language due to damage of the speech and language centers of the brain.

Aphonia: Loss of the ability to vibrate the vocal cords to produce voice. The complete lack of phonation; without voice.

Apraxia of speech: Loss of the ability to conceptualize, plan, and sequence motor speech due to a neurological disorder; verbal apraxia.

Aprosody: Loss of the rhythm and melody of speech.

Arousal: Increased awareness of and responsiveness to internal and external stimuli.

Articulation: Shaping compressed air from the lungs into individual speech sounds. The act of moving the vocal tract structures in such a manner that speech sounds are produced.

Association: The internalization of information and the process of making it personally relevant; relating of experiences, perceptions, and thoughts.

Ataxic dysarthria: A subtype of dysarthria associated with damage to the cerebellum and the tracts leading to and from it.

Auditory-acoustic agnosia: The inability to perceive differences in speech and environmental signals; the inability to perceive salient auditory features.

Auditory closure: The process by which auditory stimuli are integrated into a perceptual whole.

Auditory discrimination: The ability to perceive differences in sounds.

Autistic fantasy: A form of escape through daydreaming, and a symbolic way of meeting psychological needs.

Body image: Awareness of one's own body; a composite vision of oneself.

Brain-mind Leap: The scientific and philosophical process of projecting the neurological activity in the brain and nervous system to what occurs in a person's mind.

Broca's area: The part of the brain largely responsible for expressive communication located in the frontal lobe in the dominant cerebral hemisphere. The cortical area associated with expressive language and motor speech production.

Catastrophic reaction: In patients with aphasia this is a psycho-biological breakdown resulting from excessive stimulation, frustration, and anxiety. It is a sudden overwhelming feeling of anxiety and the reaction to it.

Cerebral vascular accident (CVA): A disruption of the flow of blood to the brain; a stroke.

Cerebral dominance: Tendency for one cerebral hemisphere to be dominant over the other for a specific function.

Circumlocution: The substitution of a word to avoid a feared one; rearranging or rephrasing the original thought. Using a substitute word for the one that cannot be remembered or spoken.

Closed-head injury (CHI): Cerebral trauma of the non-penetrating type.

Cognition: Mental functions which include reasoning and higher order information processing. The mental processes of thinking and judgment.

Compulsivity: Unwanted, recurring urges to perform an act.

Confabulation: Giving answers to questions with no regard for their truthfulness; making up false stories.

Connotation: In addition to what the word denotes, the affective and evaluative associations made by the speaker or listener.

Consciousness: Awareness of the self and the environment.

Consummation of communication: The satisfactory completion of a speech act.

Conversion: Somatization of an emotional conflict and resulting disorder.

Conversion aphonia: Loss of voice resulting from psychic trauma; psychogenic aphonia.

Conversion deafness: Deafness resulting from psychic trauma; psychogenic deafness.

Coping styles: Habitual methods of adjusting to anxiety, stress, and unwanted changes.

Coprolalia: Unprovoked use of obscene or profane language; excessive swearing.

Decode: The process of breaking down and analyzing a signal, such as speech and language, into its component parts.

Deep agraphia: A problem with written semantic errors and poor phoneme-to-grapheme conversion.

Defense mechanisms: Conscious or subconscious thought processes and behaviors used to avoid anxiety; coping styles.

Dementia: Generalized cognitive deterioration including disorientation, impaired judgment, and memory defects; generalized intellectual deficits.

Denial: Refusal to perceive and recognize threatening, unpleasant, and intolerable realities.

Denotation: The objective referent for a word.

Depersonalization: The disruption and disintegration of one's self-concept.

Derealization: A psychological defense mechanism and coping style involving a person perceiving the world as not being real.

Disorientation: Inaccurate judgments about time, place, person, and/or situation.

Descriptive gesture: The speaker using facial, arm, and hand gestures to provide direction or explain an action.

Displacement: Shift of emotion to a neutral or less threatening person or object.

Dissociation: Separation and compartmentalizing of a person's consciousness or identity to minimize anxiety.

Dys-: A prefix indicating impaired, faulty, or deficient.

Dysarthrias: A group of neuromuscular speech disorders. Impaired speech due to neurological and/or muscular deficits

Dysfluency: An interruption in the flow of speech marked by repetitions, prolongations hesitations, or blocks. A breakdown in the rhythm of speech.

Dyskinesia: Abnormal voluntary movements.

Dystonia: Abnormal, involuntary rhythmic twisting of body structure.

Echolalia: The repetition of that which has recently been spoken. Automatically repeating or "parroting" something which has been heard.

Ego: One of the three aspects of the personality, which is involved in evaluating, directing, and controlling actions in response to reality.

Ego weakness: Reduced strength of the aspect of the personality involved in evaluating, directing, and controlling actions in response to reality.

Ego restriction: A type of avoidance where a person abandons an activity in response to anxiety; narrowing of self-involvement.

Egocentric: Self-centered.

Embolism: A mass obstructing a blood vessel that develops in one part of the vascular system and ends up in another.

Emotional lability: The involuntary exaggerated emotionality seen in some patients with neurogenic communication disorders.

Empathy: Recognition and understanding of the emotional state of another person.

Encode: The process of putting an idea or thought into a signal system, such as speech and language.

Etiology: The cause of something.

Euphoria: A heightened sense of well-being.

Executive function: Cognitive skills involved in planning, organization, executing, and monitoring complex behaviors.

Expressive language: The use of conventional encoded symbols to communicate spoken, gestured, or written concepts. Expression of the speaker's psychological state.

Expressive aphasia: A neurologically-based loss of the expressive components of speech and language: speaking, writing, and gesturing.

External frame of reference: The belief that life events are the result of chance, fate, or the actions of supernatural forces.

Extrapyramidal system: Cell nuclei and nerve fibers involved in automatic, unconscious aspects of motor coordination, posture, and movement; all of the descending pathways except those of the pyramidal system.

Facilitation: The enabling of desired behaviors, reactions, and adjustments.

Fainting: The temporary loss of consciousness due to extreme psychological distress.

Fear: The expectation of unpleasantness.

Flaccid dysarthria: A neuromuscular speech disorder associated with lower motor neuron damage.

Flaccid: A muscle that is relaxed and without tone; a weak or limp muscle.

Flat affect: Narrowed mood, emotions, and temperament; reduced subjective experience of emotion.

Fluent speech: Smooth and effortlessly produced speech without hesitations, interjections or repetitions. The act of speaking smoothly and easily.

Frame of reference: Beliefs, attitudes, and assumptions about the cause-effect of life events.

Fugue state: A rare and massive dissociation of personality resulting in the need to seek physical escape.

Functional communication: The ability to express and understand basic ideas, needs, and wants.

Gesture: Movement of the body to describe or reinforce communication.

Global agraphia: A writing impairment characterized by a limited number of correctly spelled high frequency words and a complete inability to spell nonwords.

Grammar: A general term for the rules of the form and usage of a language.

Grapheme: Printed or written symbols.

Graphemic buffer agraphia: A decay of short term writing memory, so that information about the identity and serial ordering of letters is disrupted.

Gray matter: Collection of neuronal cell bodies in the central nervous system. Gray colored tissue of the brain and spinal cord primarily made up of cell bodies.

Grief response: Predictable stages in the process of accepting unwanted change or loss.

Gustatory agnosia: A disorder relating to the perception of taste.

Gustatory: Related to the sense of taste.

Guttural: Produced in the throat; pertaining to the throat or voice.

Harshness: Voice quality caused by excessive force of vocal cord vibration. Acoustic qualities associated with hypertension of the vocal folds.

hemipariesis: A weakness of the muscles on one side of the body.

Hemiplegia: Paralysis of one half of the body.

Hemorrhage: Rupture and escape of blood from a vein or artery.

Hesitations: Unusually long pauses during speech.

Hippocampus: A structure located in the brain which plays a role in learning and memory.

Homonymous hemianopsia: Defective vision in one half of the fields of both eyes. A disorder where the patient's visual field is limited to one half of his or her total visual world.

Hostility: Chronic, antagonistic attitude or feeling.

Hyper-: Prefix meaning "too much."

Hyperkinesia: A disorder characterized by excessive, uncontrolled movements.

Hypo-: Prefix meaning too little.

Hypokinesia: Slow or diminished movements.

Hysterical aphonia: Loss of voice occurring because of psychogenic factors.

Hysterical deafness: Loss of hearing because of psychogenic factors.

Hysterical stuttering: Stuttering occurring because of psychogenic factors. Usually late onset stuttering often caused by extreme anxiety.

Id: One of the three aspects of the personality. The unconscious part of the psyche containing instinctual drives.

Ideational apraxia: Disruption of the ability to conceptualize and program a motor impulse.

Idioglossia: A distinct language invented and spoken by only one person or very few people.

Image: A mental representation of some aspect of reality.

Infarct: The sudden death of tissue because of a lack of blood supply.

Inspiration: During breathing, the process of taking air into the lungs.

Intellectualization: Excessive reasoning to avoid negative emotions; the use of reasoning to negate emotional stress.

Intelligence: The ability to reason, problem solve, acquire, and retain knowledge.

Intelligibility: The ability to be understood by a listener; usually measured in percent.

Internal monologue: Communicating with one's self; self-talk or inner speech.

Internal frame of reference: The belief that one can influence or control the outcome of events.

Ischemic: Inadequate flow of blood to a part of the body.

Jargon: Fluent, but unintelligible speech; fluent speech that makes no sense.

Jargon aphasia: A type of aphasia where the patient utters fluent speech but it makes little or no sense.

Kinesthesia: The perception of one's body movement. In speech, the perception of movement and direction of the speech musculature.

Language: The multimodal ability to encode, decode, and manipulate symbols for the purposes of verbal thought or communication. Rule governed, socially shared code for representing concepts through the use of symbols.

Limbic system: A group of interconnected structures involving emotion, memory, and learning.

Linguistic competence: The knowledge of language codes.

Linguistic performance: The use of language in everyday conversation, the user's actual use of language.

Linguistic regression theory: The theory that aphasia is a regression in linguistic and cognitive functioning.

Localization: In neurology, the identification of areas of the brain responsible for specific aspects of physical, mental, or emotional functioning.

Logorrhea: Continuous fluent incoherent production of words.

Lower motor neurons: Motor neurons below the synapse.

Metacognition: Mental executive function of being aware of one's own thought processes; thinking about thinking.

Metastasis: Migration and spreading of a disease from one location to another.

Mitigated echolalia: When a person repeats the last thing spoken by someone else when bidding for time to process information.

Mixed dysarthria: Two or more dysarthrias occurring concurrently, or the changing of dysarthria type over time.

Modality: Any avenue or mode of communication.

Morpheme: The smallest unit of meaning in language; minimal unit of speech that is meaningful.

Motor speech disorders: Pertaining to disorders of motor tracts and muscles; apraxia of speech and the dysarthrias.

Multiple personalities: Two or more distinct personalities within the same individual.

Mutism: Completely without speech; inability to phonate and articulate.

Neologism: A made-up or invented word. A conventional word used in an unconventional manner.

Neuroscience: The interdisciplinary science which studies the brain, emotions, and behaviors.

Nonfluency: The absence of fluent speech.

Nonverbal communication: Communication without using spoken words.

Obsessive-compulsive: Persistent adherence to thoughts and beliefs, and the need to perform certain rituals to excess.

Olfactory: Related to the sense of smell.

Olfactory agnosia: A disorder relating to the perception of odors.

Oral apraxia: Loss of the ability to conceptualize, plan, and sequence voluntary oral nonspeech movements due to a neurological disorder.

Orientation: Awareness of time, place, person, and situation.

Palsy: Paresis or paralysis of a muscle.

Paraphasia: An aphasic naming disorder characterized by choosing the incorrect word, which either rhymes or has a semantic relationship to the correct one; literal and verbal paraphasias.

Passive-aggression: The indirect expression of anger, aggression, and hostility by the use of procrastination, lying, making excuses, complaining, and other passive actions and behaviors.

Perception: Realizing the significance of sensory information; awareness and appreciation of the salient aspects of a stimulus. Organization and interpretation of incoming sensory information.

Perseveration: The automatic continuation of a speaking or writing response that is seen in some patients with aphasia. Sensory and motor responses which persist for a longer duration than what would be warranted by the intensity and significance of the stimuli.

Phobia: Excessive and abnormal fear.

Phonation: Any voiced sound that occurs at the level of the vocal cords. Transformation of acoustic energy within the larynx by means of vocal fold vibration.

Phonatory apraxia: Loss of the ability to conceptualize, plan, and sequence voluntary laryngeal movements due to a neurological disorder.

Phonetics: The study of the acoustics, perception, classification, description, and production of speech sounds of a language.

Phonology: The study of the sounds of a language, and the way they are combined into words; the study of the sound system of a language.

Primary progressive aphasia: Degenerative brain condition where language becomes slowly and progressively impaired while other cognitive functions are preserved.

Pragmatics: The social use of language; social communicative functions and abilities.

Prognosis: A prediction about how well a patient will recover from a disease, disorder, or disability.

Projection: Attributing one's own intolerable wishes, thoughts, motivations, and feelings to another person.

Propositionality: The meaningfulness and amount of content in an utterance.

Prosody: Patterns of speech such as stress, intonation, rhythm, melody, and pitch.

Psychoacoustics: Study of psychological responses to sound.

Psychogenic: Of emotional or affective origin.

Psychology: The study of human consciousness; methods of measuring, explaining and changing behavior in humans and other animals.

Quadriplegia: Paralysis or weakness of all four extremities.

Quality-of-life: A combination of factors that contribute to satisfaction with life.

Rationalization: The attempt to justify or make acceptable intolerable feelings, behaviors, and motives.

Reaction formation: Avoidance of anxiety by engaging in thoughts and behaviors which are opposite of what one would really like to do.

Receptive aphasia: A neurologically-based loss of the receptive components of language: auditory comprehension, reading, and gesturing.

Receptive language: The use of conventional decoded symbols to understand phonemes, words, gestures, and graphemes.

Referent: The aspect of reality referred to by the symbol.

Regression: In psychology, the retreat to an earlier and more comfortable level of development and adjustment due to stress.

Rehabilitation: Therapeutic restoration of a deficient function, such as communication, to normal or near-normal levels.

Reinforcement: The positive or negative consequences of a behavior.

Reinforcing gestures: Gestures used to emphasize, accentuate, and stress a verbal statement.

Repression: Involuntary exclusion of a painful thought or memory from awareness.

Respiration: The act of breathing; inspiration and expiration.

Retrograde amnesia: Amnesia for events prior to an illness or traumatic injury to the brain.

Syncope: The temporary loss of consciousness; fainting.

Self-concept: Awareness of oneself particularly in relation to others; images and definitions of self.

Self-esteem: Positive belief and feelings about one's self-concept.

Semantics: The relationship between a language symbol and what it represents; the meaning of words.

Senility: Cognitive and intellectual deterioration associated with pathological aging.

Sensation: The detection of environmental stimuli involving the sense organs such as the eye, skin, and ear.

Short term memory: Temporary storage of information requiring continual rehearsal.

Somnambulism: Walking while asleep

Spastic: A form of paralysis where a muscle is contracted all of the time due to a neurological injury or disease; hypertonicity.

Spastic dysarthria: Neuromuscular speech disorder associated with upper motor lesions.

Speech act: The verbal expression of an intent; an act of propositional verbal communication.

Spontaneous recovery: The period of time post onset where the brain naturally resolves part or all of the neurogenic disorder.

Stress: Mental and emotional tension arising from fear, anxiety, conflicts, temporal urgency, and excessive stimulation.

Stroke (CVA): A sudden deprivation of blood supply to the brain.

Subcortical: The areas of the brain below the cerebral cortex.

Sublimation: Engaging in a socially acceptable substitute pattern of behavior for one which is blocked in an effort to reduce anxiety

Substitution: A defense mechanism and coping style used to reduce anxiety by disguising the motivations for doing something; a person replaces an unacceptable or unattainable goal, emotion, or motive with one that is attainable or acceptable.

Superego: One of the three aspects of the personality which is involved with values, ethics, and conscience.

Suppression: Intentional exclusion of thoughts and feelings from consciousness.

Surface agraphia: Writing typical of partial knowledge of written word forms.

Symbol: An entity that represents something else.

Syndrome: A combination or cluster of symptoms that usually occur together.

Syntax: The grammatical structure of language, especially word order.

Tactile: Relating to the sense of touch.

Tactile agnosia: Disorder relating to the perception of touch.

Tip-of-the-tongue phenomenon: Phonemic and semantic trial-and-error behaviors to find the desired and correct word.

Transient ischemic attack (TIA): Like a stroke, but does not result in permanent damage to the brain, and lasts fewer than twenty-four hours.

Telegraphic speech: Communication using a minimum of function words, and using a high number of content words; similar to a telegram.

Tremor: An oscillation or vibration of a muscle or structure of the body.

Tic: A sudden twitch; an involuntary repeated contraction of a muscle or muscle group.

Tract: Central nervous system axons having a common origin and destination; anatomically related parts of the central nervous system.

Traumatic brain injury (TBI): Injury to the brain caused by a blunt force or a penetrating object.

Undoing: A defense mechanism and coping style where there is an attempt through action or communication to take back an unacceptable behavior or thought; an attempt to atone for some word or action.

Unilateral neglect: Difficulty attending to one side of the body.

Upper motor neurons: Motor neurons above the synapse.

Ventricles: Interconnected, fluid-filled cavities in the brain.

Visual agnosia: A disorder relating to the perception of written words, forms, and objects.

Visual neglect: Lack of attention to a particular space or visual field.

Wernicke's area: The part of the left hemisphere of the brain largely responsible for receptive language; a cortical conduit to the larger processes of oral language understanding and comprehension.

Index

abstract thought, 9, 12
acceptance, 88–89, 93–95
adaptability continuum, 55
aggressiveness, 34, 48. *See also* passive-aggression
agnosias, perception and, 13–14
agraphia
    aphasic, 18–19
    deep and surface, 19
    parietal, 22
    pure, 19
alexia
    aphasic, 22–23
    deep, 22–23
    without agraphia, 23
altruism, 68–69, 75
amnesia, 62–63
    anterograde, 5
    repression and, 62
    retrograde, 5, 49, 63, 69
anger
    avoiding contributing to, 96–97
    in grieving, 90–92
anosognosia, 43–44, 45, 50
antidepressants, 42–43
anxiety disorders, 40. *See also* depression-anxiety disorder
apathy, 48
aphasia

anterior, 16
classifying, 14–16
defining, 5–7
desolation of, 2
etiology of, 3–5
apraxia of speech, 1, 4–6, 8, 14–18, 24, 30, 64
association school of thought, 11
attentiveness, increased or decreased, 48, 90
auditory comprehension disorders, 20–21
auditory neural impulses, 20
autistic fantasy, 58–59, 60
autistic surrender, 68
avoidance, 55–56, 60, 76
awareness, disorders of, 5, 69, 72, 75, 82

bargaining, 90–92, 97
behavioral competence, 28
blindsight phenomenon, 45
brain
    advanced techniques for studying, 13
    auditory areas of, 20–21
    blood supply to, 3
    function localization in, 10–11
    mapping of, 14–15
    psychology of aphasia and, 10–13
    speech and language areas of, 14–15
    tumors of, 4
    Wernicke's area, 20–21, 35, 36

Printed in the United States
by Baker & Taylor Publisher Services

Printed in the United States
by Baker & Taylor Publisher Services